Praise for *Living Well with Dr. Michelle*

"*Living Well with Dr. Michelle* is an essential read for holistic health! You'll find yourself more in touch with your body, in tune with your environment, and in awe of a new, sustainable well of personal energy vivacity."

—Dr. Mindy H. Pelz, *New York Times* bestselling author of *Eat Like a Girl* and *Fast Like a Girl*

"*Living Well with Dr. Michelle* is a profound guide to reclaiming health and vitality in a world where many feel overwhelmed and disconnected from their well-being. Dr. Michelle Jorgensen artfully weaves together the advancements of modern science with the enduring wisdom of holistic practices, crafting a road map that is both accessible and actionable. With her groundbreaking Cell Well model, she reveals the interconnectedness of our cellular health, empowering readers to unlock sustained energy, balanced well-being, and proactive disease prevention.

What truly distinguishes this book is its compassionate, practical approach. Dr. Michelle candidly shares her personal journey, along with deeply relatable anecdotes that underscore the transformative power of the principles she teaches. Her clear, step-by-step guidance makes even complex health concepts understandable, providing readers with the confidence to take charge of their health. Whether your goal is to overcome chronic challenges, elevate your energy, or embrace a more vibrant way of living, *Living Well with Dr. Michelle* equips you with the tools and inspiration to create lasting transformation.

This book is more than a guide—it is an invitation to rediscover the extraordinary healing potential within you. A must-read for anyone ready to take the next step toward their healthiest, most vibrant life."

—Dr. Bradley Nelson, author of *The Emotion Code*

"Dr. Michelle Jorgensen's personal and professional experience provides a unique perspective on the vital world of holistic health."

—Dr. Josh Redd, NMD, MAPHB, founder of RedRiver Health and Wellness

"Dr. Michelle is using her gifts to teach what is missing out there in the health world! I love how she combines both Eastern and Western medicine to get the best of all things healing. Reading this will leave you inspired and uplifted knowing that change is possible because nature offers all of the tools you need to feel well!"

—Karalynne Call, founder of Just Ingredients

"Dr. Michelle's simple lifestyle changes—to nutrition, breathing, your environment, exposure to toxins, and more—will have a profound impact on the whole-body ecosystem, allowing you to ditch fatigue and become the most vibrant version of yourself."

—Richie Norton, bestselling author of *Anti-Time Management*

"For anyone struggling with stress or fatigue, *Living Well with Dr. Michelle* will help you reconnect with your body, detoxify your life, and discover an untapped reservoir of energy and health. Everything in her book comes from real, raw, personal experience."

—Robyn Openshaw, MSW, 16-time author and
founder of GreenSmoothieGirl.com

"*Living Well with Dr. Michelle* is a masterful guide to understanding and nurturing your health at its core—the cellular level. Dr. Michelle's expertise as a holistic dentist and traditional naturopath shines through in this accessible, practical, and enlightening book. By bridging natural wisdom with modern science, she demystifies the complexities of wellness and provides readers with actionable tools to create lasting health."

—Dr. Caitlin Czezowski, DC, CFMP, CACCP, creator of Doc.Talks.Detox

"Dr. Michelle takes cutting-edge wellness science and makes it easy and practical for everyone to implement in their daily lives. I loved the easy-to-read stories that also taught valuable lessons. This is an accessible and empowering book. Highly recommended."

—Marjory Wildcraft, founder of The Grow Network
and author of *The Grow System*

Living Well

with Dr. Michelle

Also by Michelle Jorgensen

Healthy Mouth, Healthy YOU

Be Prepared, Not Scared

Self-Sufficient Living

100 Days From the Garden

Real Food for Real Families

Living Well

with Dr. Michelle

A Comprehensive Handbook
for Optimal Health and
Unlimited Energy

Michelle Jorgensen, DDS

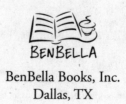

BenBella Books, Inc.
Dallas, TX

BenBella Books, Inc.
8080 N. Central Expressway
Suite 1700
Dallas, TX 75206
benbellabooks.com
Send feedback to feedback@benbellabooks.com

BenBella is a federally registered trademark.

Printed in the United States of America
10 9 8 7 6 5 4 3 2 1

Library of Congress Control Number: 2024055246
ISBN 9781637746783 (hardcover)
ISBN 9781637746790 (electronic)

Editing by Karyn Ross and Greg Brown
Copyediting by Leah Baxter
Proofreading by Jenny Bridges and Becky Maines
Indexing by WordCo Indexing Services, Inc.
Illustrations by Ruth and Finn Evans
Text design and composition by PerfecType, Nashville, TN
Cover design by Morgan Carr
Printed by Lake Book Manufacturing

For everyone who wants to reclaim the ability to Live Well . . .

And for Steve, Jens, Brooklyn, Mira, Cohen, Josh, Luke, and Liza, who put up with my unique kind of crazy. Thank you for your patience when I disappear for long stretches of studying and writing. I love you all eternally!

CONTENTS

INTRODUCTION
Let There Be Light

Imagine living in a time when the world was enveloped in darkness after sunset.

People rushed to finish everything they needed to do before nightfall, knowing that after dark they'd have to rely on candles or gas lamps for dim glimmers of light. As the nineteenth century came to an end, the world was still shrouded in darkness for half of the day, but it was on the verge of a revolutionary breakthrough thanks to the ingenuity of three inventors.

In his laboratories in Menlo Park, New Jersey, Thomas Edison had embarked on a quest to unlock the secrets of electric lighting. He was working to direct the flow of electricity through a thin fiber called a filament until it heated up enough to glow. After years of experiments, his workshop lit up with the warm glow of the first incandescent light bulb. Across the Atlantic, in the quiet English countryside, Joseph Swan was navigating a similar journey of discovery. Unbeknownst to Edison, Swan had also begun to brighten the world with his own version of the electric lamp. Edison's bulbs bathed the streets of New York City in light, while Swan's lamps lit the halls of England's finest estates. This ignited a change that would illuminate the world in ways that were previously unimaginable. Suddenly, cities didn't need to sleep when the sun set. Streets gleamed with the steady brightness of electric lamps, casting away shadows and ushering in a new era of life after dark.

But the change wasn't just mechanical; it was about possibility. With the flick of a switch, work could continue long after sunset, extending productivity and reshaping the very concept of time. Factories hummed with activity, streets buzzed with life, and cities transformed into the twenty-four-seven bustling metropolises "that never sleep" that we're familiar with today.

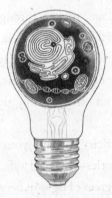

The light bulb was more than just a source of illumination; it was a catalyst for progress.

The invention of the light bulb sparked the creation of electrical grids, distribution networks, and power plants, all crucial parts of modern infrastructure. Urban planners reimagined cityscapes, designing streets filled with light and transforming once-dark alleys into vibrant thoroughfares. The light bulb's invention fueled other types of technological innovation as well, inspiring inventors and scientists to push the boundaries of possibility.

One of these inventors, Nikola Tesla, was an enigmatic visionary with a flair for the dramatic. Tesla envisioned a world where electric light could move beyond the binary of "on" or "off." His work led to the creation of the dimmer switch, which allowed a light bulb to be brightened or dimmed, depending on the amount of electricity flowing from the switch to the bulb.

The Body Electric

These innovations quite literally changed how we see the world. But did you know that your body works in ways that are strikingly similar to those darkness-shattering bulbs?

Your life depends on the flow of electricity, specifically the flow of electrons, through each cell in your body. In this book, you'll learn about this concept of "cellular" or "biologic" electricity ("bioelectricity")—the literal electrons that course through your cells and body. Think of bioelectricity as the body's own language, spoken through tiny electrical impulses. These impulses control everything from muscle movements to the beating of your heart. This is how fitness trackers today do more than just count your steps. These wearable health monitors measure the electrical activity in your heart, brain, muscles and other organs, giving you real-time insights into your health.

When this flow of electricity through your cells stops, life stops. Life and death are binary categories—on and off, light and dark. However, *living* encompasses all the degrees of light in between. Living is your miraculous body's own version of Tesla's dimmer switch. Our bodies are not simply machines designed to operate at one set speed. Instead, by adding more electrons, we can increase our energy to create the brightest, most brilliant versions of ourselves. This living is what *Living Well with Dr. Michelle* is all about.

Scientists have learned how to speak this language of bioelectricity, leading to some incredible health innovations—for example, devices called electroceuticals, which send electrical signals through your body to treat conditions like chronic pain or epilepsy. Doctors are even using electrical signals to diagnose and treat diseases by directly interacting with the nervous system, fixing what's wrong without needing medicine.

In this book, you'll discover how electrons, the workhorses of bioelectricity, power your body and influence the quality of your life. You'll also learn how you can generate more bioelectricity in your cells and how to increase your electron intake from the world around you through the earth, plants, water, and air surrounding and nourishing us.

Most importantly, you will be introduced to the Cell Well model, a natural, new, and innovative approach to wellness. Your body is made up of approximately thirty-seven trillion cells that work together, each performing specific functions to keep your body running smoothly. From red blood cells that carry oxygen to neurons that transmit signals in the brain, every cell plays a crucial role in our overall well-being. These cells live in a rich, interconnected ecosystem that never sleeps and requires constant input to keep it healthy and functioning well. Once you've learned what it takes to keep one cell in this ecosystem well, you will then be able to apply that knowledge to every cell in your body. The Cell Well model and its Elements, Seasons, and Formulas will show you how.

Understanding how cells work has opened a world of possibilities. Take stem cell therapy, for instance. Stem cells can turn into any type of cell needed, and scientists are learning to harness these cells to repair damaged tissues, offering hope for conditions like spinal injuries and heart disease. Personalized medicine is another exciting area of research. By studying an individual's genetic makeup and cellular functions, doctors can tailor treatments specifically to fit their bodies and their needs.

The *Cell Well Model*: Staying Well and Returning to Wellness

The Cell Well model has four essential divisions: Supply, Support, Secure, and Signal. To keep each cell well, you need to care for each of these divisions. And please remember, keeping one cell well is the foundation for keeping every cell well.

Step 1: Supply Essential Nutrients and Oxygen
Step 2: Support the Cellular Environment and Waste Removal
Step 3: Secure Immune Response and Detoxification
Step 4: Signal for Communication and Stress Response

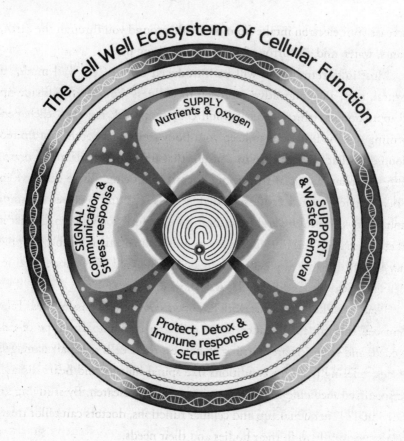

The Cell Well Ecosystem Of Cellular Function

SUPPLY
Nutrients & Oxygen

SIGNAL
Communication &
Stress response

SUPPORT
& Waste Removal

Protect, Detox &
Immune response
SECURE

Throughout *Living Well with Dr. Michelle,* you will dive deeply into this model and learn, in detail, how it works. You'll also learn how to create personalized Cell Well Formulas that you can apply to your specific health and wellness needs. Finally, you'll learn how to power up your cells so that you can live well.

Medicine is really all about knowing how your cells and body work and what to do proactively to keep them well. Instead of ignoring or covering up symptoms, you'll learn how to use those symptoms to identify the formulas your cells need to return to wellness. You won't have to invest in years of medical school or enroll in a "one-size-fits-all" diet, exercise, or self-help program to practice this medicine. When you learn how one of your cells does all its magnificent work, and what it requires to stay well, fend off disease, rebuild, and return to health when needed, then you will know what it takes for your entire body to be well.

While the Cell Well model is new, wellness—the goal of the model—is not. New parents are familiar with the idea of wellness; from the first week of their baby's life, these earnest and anxious caregivers take their child to be thoroughly checked by a doctor at well-child visits. However, the frequency of those visits slows down long before adulthood. Most teens and adults only go to the doctor when they are sick, not to stay well. Health care as we know it today is largely focused on curing an already present disease and reducing its accompanying symptoms. Like the browning leaves on your favorite houseplant, symptoms are your body's warning system, sending a signal to you that there is a problem. However, like your suffering plant, your body is already struggling by the time you experience a symptom. When your symptoms are severe enough to prompt a doctor's appointment, you are probably long past well.

More than 50 percent of U.S. citizens self-report that they aren't as well as they would like to be, and at the start of 2024, improving their health was the most common resolution people made.[1] Once people aren't well, they often look for pills and procedures to help them return to health—but that's a backward approach. The key is in focusing on proactive practices that will help them stay well in the first place. Such practices can turn their biological dimmer switches up to high and give them the energy to live their lives to the fullest.

Jeanne Calment, a feisty French woman, had a dimmer switch that was always on high. Born in 1875, in Arles, France, Calment lived to the ripe old age of 122 years and 164 days, passing away in 1997. She still holds the record for the longest confirmed human lifespan.

What makes Calment's story so fascinating isn't just her exceptional age, but how she lived life. Despite living through two world wars, the rise and fall of empires, and immense societal changes, Calment maintained a positive outlook and attributed her longevity to several factors. First, she stayed physically active throughout her life, cycling, swimming, and even fencing until well into her eighties. Second, she enjoyed delicious food that gave her body the nutrients she needed. She ate meals rich in olive oil, fruits, and vegetables, and even indulged in dark chocolate and occasionally port wine. Third, Calment possessed a remarkable sense of humor and resilience that served her well through life's ups and downs. Her sharp wit and positive attitude endeared her to people around the world.

Calment's longevity not only made her a celebrity in her later years, but also sparked scientific interest in understanding the secrets to living a long and healthy life. Were the secrets genetic, lifestyle-related, environmental, or a combination? In the coming chapters, we'll use the latest science, traditional wisdom, and plain common sense to investigate and answer these questions.

Being sick was what started my quest for better health and wellness. Maybe being sick is what has brought you to these pages, too. But Calment's story shows that you don't have to get sick before working on wellness. It can be a cultivated, lifelong practice, ensuring that you don't have to droop, wilt, or struggle, even later in life.

Get Ready to Turn Your Dimmer Switch to High

It's much easier to stay well than it is to regain health that you've lost. But what is wellness? What is health? What is disease? When do you cross the threshold between them?

Let's start by defining terms we will use throughout the book:

+ **Health** is the level of a person's physical and mental soundness in the absence of disease.
+ **Diseases** are abnormalities in the function and/or structure of organs and systems in the body.
+ **Lifespan** is the total length of life, regardless of the quality of health and wellness during that time.
+ **Healthspan** is the total duration of time a person enjoys good health and well-being, without impaired daily functioning.

+ **Medicine** is the knowledge, skills, practices, and substances used to maintain and restore health, treat illness, and improve lifespan and healthspan.
+ **Wellness** goes beyond health, and is much more than the physical absence of disease. It refers to the state of overall well-being that includes physical, mental, emotional, social, and spiritual wholeness.

Wellness means that you have the energy you need to live your life to its full potential.

Like Jeanne Calment, you can turn your dimmer switch on life up to high. In Part One of *Living Well with Dr. Michelle*, through my story and others, you will learn how cells work, what they need to be well, and how to deal with health challenges we as humans all face. You will also learn how people in generations past stayed well and lived well and how to combine that with modern medical knowledge to supercharge your cells and energy. Part Two will dive into the natural and freely available secrets to wellness that the modern world seems to have forgotten, secrets that are found in nature's Five Elements (fire, plants, earth, air, and water). You'll learn when your cells need the support of each Element and you'll explore practical and actionable ways to use the Elements to energize and strengthen your body's cells. Finally, in Part Three, you will take the Seasons of Wellness Assessment to determine the starting point of your personalized wellness journey. You will learn how to use the Cell Well model to re-energize your life and take control of your health, healthspan, and wellness. This section is capped off with recipes, exercises, products, and recommendations to help you really live well.

On your way through the *Living Well with Dr. Michelle* journey, you'll be introduced to breakthroughs in history and science, combining innovative modern medicine with knowledge and wisdom from wrinkled grandmothers and wise healers of the past. You'll also be introduced to people I've helped—you may see yourself in their stories.

I want to help you live well every day, do what you love, and fulfill your unique potential. That potential is dependent on learning how to power up your cells, find health and healing everywhere around you, and live with unbelievable levels of energy, naturally. It's possible. You are the one with your finger on your own dimmer switch. Everything you need to know to live your life to its fullest and reach your highest potential is right here in these pages.

Let's get started.

All resources in *Living Well with Dr. Michelle* can be found at www.resources.livingwellbook.com. This is your go-to place for access to all the Assessments, Guides, recipes, resources, and recommendations. Check in frequently to stay up to date.

PART ONE

Foundations of Wellness

CHAPTER 1

....

Wellness Misunderstood

Jack LaLanne, the legendary "Godfather of Fitness," was an icon of health and wellness, but you might be surprised to find out that he didn't start out that way. Born in San Francisco in 1914, LaLanne wrestled with poor health as a child and was a self-described "sugarholic" and "junk food junkie" until he was fifteen years old. His life took a dramatic turn for the better after listening to a public lecture about the benefits of good nutrition by health food pioneer Paul Bragg, which ignited a fire in LaLanne.

Determined to overhaul his lifestyle, LaLanne dove headfirst into a world of physical fitness and nutrition. He started lifting weights at a time when that was nearly unheard of, and at the age of twenty-one, he set up the nation's first modern health studio in Oakland, California. His pioneering wellness innovations extended into the field of nutrition, where he popularized juicing, protein bars, and supplements. However, it was LaLanne's groundbreaking television show, *The Jack LaLanne Show*, that catapulted him, and his ideas about health and fitness, into the national spotlight. For more than three decades, LaLanne graced television screens across America, demonstrating exercises and preaching the gospel of healthy living with infectious enthusiasm.

LaLanne's success wasn't just confined to the small screen. He was a real-life action hero, shattering records and defying age-based expectations of performance with jaw-dropping feats of strength and endurance. At sixty, he stunned the world by swimming from Alcatraz Island to Fisherman's Wharf in San Francisco while shackled, handcuffed, and towing a one thousand–pound boat. This swim is approximately 1.25 miles (two kilometers), a distance made even more challenging by the area's strong currents and cold temperatures, as well as the potential presence of great white sharks. In addition to swimming stunts like this, LaLanne set records for the most push-ups and pull-ups performed in a single session by a senior citizen, proving that age was merely a number to be defied.

But LaLanne wasn't just about pumping iron and breaking records. He was a beacon of vitality and inspiration, reminding his followers and the general public that with passion and perseverance, anything is possible. A visionary who believed in the boundless potential that lies within each of us, and who championed preventive health care and healthy aging long before it became mainstream, LaLanne came to believe that the country's overall health depended on the health of its population, referring to physical culture and nutrition as "the salvation of America."[2] When he passed away in 2011 at the age of ninety-six, LaLanne left behind a legacy that continues to inspire millions to prioritize their health and wellness.

Wellness Is Already Inside of You

You and I have one very important thing in common with this wellness legend: each of us has been given one amazing, miraculous body to live in for our travels through this life.

Did you know that your brain can hold five times as much information as the *Encyclopedia Britannica*,[3] and that your nerve impulses travel at 170 miles per hour on the same amount of power as a ten-watt light bulb?[4] Or that your life-giving heart creates enough pressure to project blood thirty feet? How about the fact that in one day that blood travels a total of twelve thousand miles?[5] Not to be outdone, your eyes take in more information than the largest existing telescope; your lungs have a surface area the size of a tennis court; and you can have two-thirds of your liver removed from trauma or surgery, and it will grow back to its original size in four weeks![6] Your body is constantly repairing and rebuilding, producing three hundred billion new cells every day, all without you needing to consciously direct the process.[7]

This incredible body is made up of approximately thirty-seven trillion tiny little packages called cells. Our cells are the basic building blocks of our amazing bodies, and they have a breathtaking capacity to self-heal and regenerate. Remember the last time you cut your finger? It probably hurt for a few minutes, was sore for a day or two, then you stopped thinking about it. You may have covered it with a bandage, but the bandage didn't heal your finger. It was your body and its cells that helped the two sides of the cut grow together and make scar tissue strong enough that the skin would not separate again. If you break a bone, a doctor may set it, but it is your body that knits the bone together and makes it like new. If you get a bacterial infection, you may take an antibiotic to kill the bacteria, but your body must sweep the area free of infection, clean up the mess, and replace the damaged cells.

When we think about wellness from a cellular standpoint, we see that healing and wellness are already inside of us, that we embody these principles simply through the fact that our body, if properly supported, works with single-minded effort to return to a state of wellness. In the current paradigm of Western medicine, pills and medical treatments are often life-savers, providing essential support when our bodies need a helping hand. However, a common misunderstanding about advances in medicine today is that those prescriptions and procedures are healing your body. In reality, their role is to boost our natural healing processes, not take over the job entirely. Your cells are the ones doing the work, and at times, are grateful for the support and help Western or traditional medicine can provide.

The truth is that when you give your cells what they need to stay well in the first place, you don't need healing at all. And if a part of your body becomes unwell, either due to disease or lifestyle stressors, there's often a path back to health that's again rooted in our bodies and the world around us.

Wellness Defined

We are bombarded with a confusing mix of messages about wellness, health, medicine, and healing. Media, advertisements, search engines, and well-meaning friends and family fill your feed and mind with their version of each one. It seems like every day someone starts up a new podcast sharing tips and advice on how to live a healthier life.

But what does all this advice mean? What's accurate and what's not? Where should you even start?

There are so many different opinions, approaches, and products that it's virtually impossible to read, listen to, and understand all that's being shared. If you have a cough and go to the internet or social media right now, you'll find these suggestions and more:

> Drink plenty of water . . . Eat a spoonful of honey . . . Have some herbal tea . . . Gargle with salt water . . . Eat a slice of pineapple . . . Reduce inflammation with ginger . . . Have a warm turmeric drink . . . Add probiotics to your diet . . . and finally . . . Take an over-the-counter cough medicine!

Do any of these "medicines" actually help "cure" a cough? Perhaps. But using them may also lead to more questions than answers. How much should I use? How often? Is this medicine covering up the cough or helping correct the reason for the cough? And what is it doing to my body and cells?

It seems that there's an equally long and confusing list of recommendations online for every worrisome symptom you could possibly experience. In our media- and information-saturated world, there is a pill, powder, or prescription for everything, but I've found from listening to the questions of my patients and social media followers that these "clickbait" answers and recommendations tend to leave people more confused—and no closer to wellness.

If I asked you to give me your definition of medicine, what would you say? Would your family, friends, and neighbors give the same definition?

I sent an informal survey to 150,000 followers on social media to learn how people define medicine today and found that almost everyone was looking at it in a different way. The survey results fell into three broad categories. First, some cynically described medicine as "something scary that doesn't really help," "artificial substances that mask symptoms," and "sick care." Others took a more positive view of medicine, explaining it as "a protocol to eliminate disease" and "anything that brings you back to wholeness." A third group attributed the term "medicine" to things like laughter, food, herbs, oils, sunlight, vitamins, and prescription medications.

With so many types of medicine in the world, shouldn't we be the healthiest, happiest people that have ever lived on the planet? Well, we aren't. Although per capita health spending increased in every first-world country in the last few years,[8] a poll conducted in 2023 found that 54 percent of Americans think the current health-care system is going in the wrong direction. Nearly three-quarters of U.S. adults say that the health-care system is not meeting their needs in some way, and some respondents even went as far as to say the system gets in the way of them receiving the care they need.[9]

Unfortunately, it seems those respondents are correct. For the second year in a row, life expectancy in the United States has dropped. It is currently at 76.1 years, its lowest level since 1996.[10] True, that statistic has been impacted by the COVID-19 pandemic, but life expectancy in the U.S., even before the pandemic, had been growing at a slightly slower curve than overall world life expectancy.[11] Even more telling is the current average "healthspan." Healthspan—the period during which a person is generally healthy and free from serious illnesses like diabetes, arthritis, and heart disease—is a measure of your *quality of life,* and it's all about having the energy to live the life you want.

Healthspan and lifespan estimates for people in the US and worldwide in 2021:[12]

+ Global lifespan: 71.4 years
+ Global healthspan: 61.9 years

These figures indicate that while people are living longer, the number of years lived without significant health issues is dropping. An adult in the world today can expect to live to the age of 71.4, but their body and mind may only function well (or, their healthspan will last) for 61.9 of those years. That means that, statistically, anyone nearing their early-sixties might expect their last full decade of life to be spent in suboptimal health without the energy to do what they want. More than 9.5 million seniors in the United States[13] live for some period in long-term care facilities, designed for older adults who need help with activities such as bathing, eating, dressing, or moving from a bed to a chair.[14] These are all activities most hope to be able to do for themselves long past their mid-sixties! The fact that this industry is booming is evidence that today's older generation is living longer but not living well.[15]

Unfortunately, things are not looking better for future generations either. Science is finding that the types of disease, and the number of people suffering from them, have increased among younger generations.[16] For the first time in recorded history, children are sicker than their parents and grandparents were at the same age.[17] Comparing the health of younger generations to their grandparents is a complex process influenced by various factors such as advancements in health care, changes in lifestyle, diet, environmental factors, and diagnostic criteria. However, some trends already suggest that younger generations may look forward to specific health challenges. Particularly in developed countries, young people are experiencing higher rates of obesity compared to previous generations. According to the World Health Organization, obesity rates have nearly doubled since 1990,[18] which is concerning because obesity is associated with various health issues such as type 2 diabetes, cardiovascular diseases, and certain cancers.[19] Younger generations are also facing an increased burden of chronic diseases such as autoimmune conditions, allergies, mental health conditions, and asthma.[20] While improved diagnostics may contribute to higher reported rates, changes in lifestyle habits including excessive screen time, reduced physical activity, increased consumption of processed foods and sugary beverages, and lower intake of fruits, vegetables, and other nutrient-dense foods could also be affecting these trends. People of younger generations are also growing up in environments with increased pollution, exposure to chemicals, and climate change-related challenges.[21, 22] All of these changes have significantly affected mental health, with levels of stress, anxiety, depression, and other mental health disorders on the rise.[23]

The data presents a bleak prospect of our children's future and leads to some big questions. When much of medical technology has leaped forward, why are there so many negative trends? Why do we seem to be taking so many steps backward?

For the most part, life expectancy has steadily increased since 1900, when the average American lived only 47 years.[24] During that era, living conditions were characterized by widespread air, water, and food pollution. Cities were plagued with unsanitary conditions, leading to rampant outbreaks of diseases such as whooping cough, diphtheria, tuberculosis, and measles, which claimed countless lives due to limited medical knowledge. Since then, a combination of health regulations, advancements in food production and safety, improvements in sanitation, and medical breakthroughs have extended the average lifespan by three decades. Some of these transformative changes were driven by the tireless efforts of medical pioneers, like:

- ✦ Dr. Sara Josephine Baker, who tackled the problem of infant mortality.[25]
- ✦ Drs. Grace Eldering and Pearl Kendrick and chemist Loney Gordon, who worked tirelessly to develop a whooping cough vaccine.[26]
- ✦ Social reformer Jane Addams, who cleaned up dirty, disease-ridden streets.[27]
- ✦ Progressive novelist Upton Sinclair, whose exposé *The Jungle* prompted reforms in the meatpacking industry.[28]
- ✦ Nathan Straus, part owner of Macy's department store, who established pasteurization stations to provide safe milk to children.[29]
- ✦ And more . . .

Where and how have our continual advances in quality of life and health been derailed? Those are the questions scientists and medical providers are scrambling to answer.

Many infectious diseases that once were sure to kill or disable have been nearly eradicated; babies and mommas are much safer in childbirth; and if you break an arm or slice open your head, you will quickly, efficiently, and effectively get patched up and sent on your way home to heal. This is the kind of medicine that has improved exponentially since the 1900s, and it is the kind of medicine that repairs and saves lives. You know it as "modern medicine," and it's research- and science-driven.

However, many people today have changed their thinking about what medicine should do for them. Modern medicine is largely applied for the care of disease or emergencies rather than on things that keep you well and prevent everyday illnesses and chronic disease in the first place. Setting a broken bone or recovering from a heart attack or stroke is best taken care of by a physician in a hospital. There is no debate about that. Because of the amazing work that doctors, nurses, pharmacists, and others do in these situations, people today have largely outsourced all their health care to modern medical practitioners, and the work of those practitioners is unparalleled in keeping you alive. But as the studies about healthspan show,[30] this is not the medicine that proactively helps your body, or you, stay well.

Kate, one of my most fragile patients, knew all about not staying well. She had been a successful therapist with her own thriving practice, but she hadn't been able to work in two years. The day I met her, she was rail thin with sparse gray hair that barely hid her scalp. Despite eating well over 3,000 calories a day (1,000 calories more than a typical adult woman), she was losing weight because of chronic, debilitating diarrhea. Nothing she ate stayed in her system, and she felt like she was in an all-out war with her body. Living with a miserable quality of life and rarely leaving the house, Kate was desperate for answers. Her problems made no sense to her or her health-care providers because she was doing everything that they instructed her to do, and more. The problem was that those providers were treating her symptoms but missing the root cause. To find that root cause, Kate needed to discover and understand what was negatively affecting her body.

That answer lay in the inner workings of her cells.

Cells Discovered

Early in the seventeenth century, the world was buzzing with curiosity about the nature of life. It was a time when the microscopic realm of the world and the human body remained hidden from human eyes and understanding. Enter Robert Hooke, a true Renaissance man. Hooke was a sickly child, born in 1635 on a windswept island off the southern coast of England. His father died when he was thirteen, prompting Hooke to leave home and start studying at Westminster School in London. He had an inheritance of one hundred pounds in his pocket and an infinitely long list of questions about science and life in his head. Driven by insatiable curiosity, Hooke constantly pushed the boundaries of knowledge. His curiosity took him from Westminster School to the laboratories of Oxford back to the bustling city of London, where he became the first curator of experiments at the Royal Society, the country's preeminent scientific academy.

While in this position, Hooke studied the work of ancient scientists. He was unsettled to find that many of their theories had remained unquestioned for centuries. Looking for ways to improve on the scientific methods of the day, Hooke learned of a technological marvel that would change the course of scientific history: the microscope. Invented by Dutch spectacle-makers in the late sixteenth century, this optical wonder allowed scientists to peer into a previously unseen world. Scientists worked to improve these first instruments, and in the 1660s, armed with a simple yet powerful compound microscope, Hooke took a magnified look at a humble piece of cork. Upon microscopic examination, Hooke saw a network of small, box-like structures resembling the cells of a monastery. He coined the term "cell" to describe these microscopic chambers. Hooke's groundbreaking discovery more than four hundred years ago marked the birth of cell science, one of the cornerstones of modern biology. The revelation that living organisms were composed of these basic units challenged centuries-old beliefs and sparked a revolution about the understanding of life itself.[31, 32]

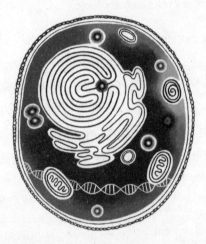

A single cell, containing the cellular ecosystem of life.

The scientific community wrestled with Hooke's findings but couldn't argue with the hidden world the microscope revealed. Uncovering the intricate ecosystem of life at the cellular level, Hooke unearthed a simple and profound truth: cells provide the structure and house the functional parts of all living things, from microorganisms to humans.

Scientists consider cells to be the smallest form of life on our planet. Where Hooke left off, other scientists took over. They discovered that cells held the biological workings that make the compounds, chemicals, and signals responsible for everything that happens inside your body.[33] Every cell is like a microscopic metropolis, where tiny structures work together to keep your cell, and your life, humming along. Your body is bustling with so much activity it makes the busiest city seem like a quiet village in comparison.

In a city, when power goes out, water lines break, or weather makes roads impassable, life as you know it turns into frustrated chaos. Similarly, when essential functions in your cells stop working as they should, your body's systems become disorganized and begin to malfunction, leading to early cell death, or worse, uncontrolled growth that Western medicine calls cancer.

A perfect example of what happens when cellular systems fail is plaque buildup in arteries. Let's take a closer look:

Phase 1: Damage: The problem starts when the endothelial cells—the cells lining the artery walls—are damaged by something inside or outside the body, like inflammation, autoimmune disease, infection, high blood pressure, or toxins like cigarette smoke, among other things.

Phase 2: Infiltration of defenses: If the damaged cells aren't repaired, the endothelial cells are unable to do their job of clearing toxins out of the arteries. They let their defenses down and allow fats, cholesterol, calcium, and toxins to build up on the artery walls, forming plaque.

Phase 3: Immune reaction: The body jumps into action, sending immune cells called macrophages to the site of injury. The macrophages attempt to remove the growing plaque but can become overwhelmed, transforming into dysfunctioning cells themselves that become part of the plaque buildup.

Phase 4: Cover-up: Over time, smooth muscle cells migrate from the middle layer of the arterial wall to the site of injury to attempt to remove the mess the other cells have left behind. The muscle cells do this by throwing a biological "tarp" of connective tissue over the areas of buildup, helping to stabilize them so they are less likely to rupture or break free and lead to a heart attack.

Phase 5: Worsened disease: This pile of dysfunctional cells covered by connective tissue then further blocks the arteries, leading to reduced blood flow and higher blood pressure. This cycle continues and contributes to the progression of the original problem, leading to new complications that we know as types of heart disease: coronary artery disease, heart attack, heart failure, heart rhythm problems like tachycardia and atrial fibrillation, heart valve disease, and more.

In your arteries and every other part of your body, disease starts with the cells. Keeping the lining cells healthy in the first place leads to arteries that are clear of plaque buildup, blood pressure that can be managed without pharmaceutical help, and no further heart complications.

Disease is simply the result of cellular dysfunction.

Modern medicine tests for disease with blood tests, biopsies, cultures, and X-rays, which give an amazing glimpse into the inner workings of your body and its cells. For example, to detect heart disease, an EKG, stress test, blood tests, or an MRI might be recommended. These technologies are marvelous. But the intrinsic problem with most modern-day testing is that it investigates problems that already exist and malfunctions that are already negatively affecting how your cells and body are functioning. By the time a deficiency or excess shows up on a blood test, you've probably been experiencing problems for some time. By the time you fail a stress test for your heart, you've already developed blockage in your arteries. This approach is about reactively responding to disease, not about proactively caring for wellness.

Disease care is doing something after the fact to help your cells and body return to correct function. Wellness is about proactively keeping your cells well in the first place.

A New Model of Wellness

Very little of what's touted as health care today is focused on keeping cells well or empowering you to preserve your own wellness—the goal at the heart of the Cell Well model. Understanding the model begins with understanding how our cells work their magic. It's time to get reintroduced to your cells and the amazing, bustling inner world that literally keeps you alive and helps you stay well.

How Cells Work: Cell Signaling to Maintain Wellness

The inner workings of your cells are intricate and efficient, with each cell and each function within the cell playing a crucial role. To function properly and optimally, each of your cells and their cellular functions require electricity. As long as your cells have that electricity, and the power doesn't go out, your body remains alive. Even while you are sleeping, your body is using energy: your brain is backing up memories, your body's construction crews are rebuilding and repairing cells, and your body's energy systems are recharging.

All your "powered-up" cells are connected to an electrical grid, which both ensures nonstop energy and provides a way for the cells to communicate with each other. This biological electrical grid is very similar to the electrical grid and power lines in a city, and the individual cells operate like individual houses connected to that grid. Each cell has its own power line, circuits, and cable or cell service bringing information in and out.

Individual cells live in bigger "neighborhoods" called organs. All the cells in an organ are similar in function and require similar inputs and services, which is why they live together in a specific area of the body. Finally, all those organ neighborhoods, together, make up the urban center that you know as your body. The electricity coursing through your body's biological electrical grid allows all your cellular, organ, and body systems to work and communicate with each other.

As you can see, there's a lot silently happening twenty-four seven in your cells. How do cells handle coordinating this massive effort? Your cells communicate by transmitting information to other cells similarly to the way humans communicate. If cells are touching each other, they can give each other a handshake or a hug. If they aren't touching, they can send up chemical signals like a signal fire or flare, electrical signals like a text message, and mechanical signals like a yell or a whisper. This type of communication, called cell signaling, is essential for life.

What does cell signaling look like in action? The last time you cut your finger, without thinking, you instinctively jerked your hand away from whatever sharp surface created the injury. That quick movement was thanks to cell signaling in your nervous system, which transmitted a message at lightning speed to your muscles. You probably noticed the red, angry swelling around the cut a day later. The redness and swelling were part of your injury alert system, where chemical signals mobilized your immune cells to protect you from infection in the cut and facilitate healing by cleaning up bacteria, dead cells, debris, and damaged tissue. As those cells in your finger encountered this stress, additional cell signaling created a cellular memory, teaching you to be more careful to avoid a cut next time. Your cut probably took around ten days to completely heal. During those days, your cells were hard at work healing the area. Using your DNA as blueprints, your cells directed the reconstruction efforts, guiding stem cells, connective tissue cells, skin cells, and more to build, repair, and regenerate tissues with meticulous precision. Your red and white blood cells, part of your lymphatic or waste system, and many of their friends, also got in on the action, their signals directing the flow of energy and nutrients to the injured tissues, fine-tuning temperature, pH, and other vitals in that cut finger so healing could happen efficiently. Together, all these actions created the optimal state for healing after the injury, and your finger got better!

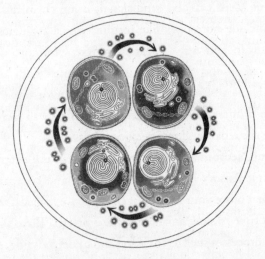

Cells communicate with each other, ensuring seamless operations of your body's organs and systems.

Cellular Communication

The transport of these cell messages outperforms any communication systems humans have created. In fact, nerve cells transmit information at speeds that would make the fastest fiber-optic cable company envious. Wellness comes from your cells and body using electrons and other chemicals and interactions to communicate. These cellular signals are the secret language of well-being your body uses to help you stay well and return to wellness when needed. This intricate network of cellular communication ensures the operation of various physiological processes, ensuring the seamless functioning of your body's diverse organs and systems. Here are a few types of cellular communication:

- **Direct:** Cells can signal each other directly when they are in physical contact with one another. Direct cell signals allow adjacent heart muscle cells to share ions quickly, enabling synchronized heartbeats. Immune cells use external proteins to activate neighboring cells during an immune response, and skin cells sense and respond to their neighbors, facilitating wound healing.

- **Chemical:** Cells can also send signals using chemicals. Chemical signals include hormones like insulin, which regulates how cells handle sugar, and neurotransmitters like serotonin, which helps regulate mood and sleep. Immune messengers such as interleukins use chemical signaling to coordinate immune responses during infection or injury. Proteins like epidermal growth factor use it to promote the repair and regeneration of tissues.

- **Electrical:** Neurons and heart and muscle cells use electrical signals to transmit sensory information like smell and taste, motor commands that move your muscles, and regulatory signals that tell you when it's time to slow down and take a breath. These signals make complex processes such as thinking and understanding, movement, and hormone regulation all possible.

- **Mechanical:** Mechanical cell signaling involves cells responding to changes in their environment. This includes blood vessel cells relaxing to allow more blood flow when they are stretched, and bone cells growing in response to physical stress and weight-bearing activities. Hair cells in the inner ear can even sense vibrations from sound waves and convert them into electrical signals, allowing you to hear.

Cellular communication ensures the seamless coordination of systems and function in your body. It is also the way your body responds to the world around you. Without the communication and energy transfer between your cells, you can't stay well.

I learned more about the crucial role cell signals play in wellness from Mark, an unlikely teacher. I first met Mark in my dental practice. When I asked what brought him to the office, he looked at the ground and confessed it had been a long time since he had visited a dentist.

He pointed to a decayed tooth that looked painful. He explained he was surfacing from a long struggle with anxiety, and at his lowest he had even thought of suicide. In this dark time, he had put off his dental care. But Mark was in my office because he wanted to get well.

The trouble had started when Mark was given an antibiotic to treat a case of strep throat. After the course of antibiotics, he was left with unexplained, life-altering anxiety. Did the antibiotic lead to his anxiety? No one seemed to know, so a second well-meaning doctor prescribed an anti-anxiety medication. This gave Mark relief from the anxiety, but then insomnia hit him like a freight train. Night after relentless night unable to fall asleep led Mark into a dark spiral of hopelessness. In a desperate attempt to find help, he began researching his situation. During those long, sleepless nights of research, Mark learned more about his cells. He came up with theories about why these medicines were affecting his health. He also discovered some possible solutions.

During Mark's dental appointment, he told me about his theories. Leaning on fuzzy memories from seventh-grade science class and a lot of Dr. Google, he had finally understood why he had stopped sleeping. The anti-anxiety medication he was given works by increasing the levels of a hormone called serotonin in the brain that regulates mood, emotions, overall well-being, and sleep. It is hypothesized that in some people with mood disorders, there is too little serotonin in the synapse to keep the mood balanced. Mark's medication caused serotonin to stay active in his brain for longer periods by blocking its reabsorption into nerve cells. However, though prolonging the action of serotonin is understood to alleviate symptoms of depression and anxiety, it can also disrupt sleep patterns and cause other side effects like dry mouth.[34] Mark's persistent insomnia was most likely the result of the medication shutting off the way his cells naturally communicated that they were tired. Simply put, Mark's brain wasn't getting the signal it needed to start the sleep cycle. And it didn't help that that bothersome dry mouth had led to plaque buildup and rapidly advancing tooth decay in his molar!

When doing his research, Mark knew he had to go back to the beginning to find a way out of the mess he was in. He knew his problems had started with strep throat, one of many stressors on his body at that time. He had never really recovered from that infection, so he concluded that his body, then and now, didn't have what it needed to heal. Again turning to Dr. Google, Mark found stories of people who had combined simple kitchen ingredients into a vitamin- and mineral-rich drink, replenishing their systems and recharging their bodies. He had nothing to lose, so he made his own concoction and started drinking it every morning. Slowly, his mood stabilized, and his sleep improved. He had the energy to face the day again.

Mark had stumbled onto a method for recharging his cells' energy and improving the way they were communicating. It sounds implausibly simple, but it's true. Mark slowly weaned himself off his anti-anxiety medicine as the flood of nutrients he drank every day gave his cells back what they needed to function properly. And, of course, Mark visited my practice to have his decayed tooth repaired and the area around it cleared of infection.

We'll get more into to specific formulas and recommendations for wellness formulas in chapters 10 and 11, but for now let's dig deeper into how Mark's drink helped his cells communicate and function as they should. Mark's drink contained three essential nutrients: vitamin C, sodium, and potassium, all of which help cells with signaling activities.

Mark's body especially needed help in his adrenal glands: small, triangular glands that sit on top of your kidneys and help you adapt to your

world and all the stressors it brings. When alerted by your cells' distress signals, the adrenals kick into high gear and start producing a rapid response
team of hormones, including cortisol and adrenaline, that prep your body
for what's coming. Think about a time you had to speak in front of a crowd
and how daunting it was. Your heartbeat accelerated, your breathing quick-
ened, your mouth went dry, and you felt a surge of energy in your muscles.
That was all thanks to your adrenal glands doing their job! When you were
done speaking and the stress was over, your adrenal glands slowed the production of stress hormones and you and all your cells started to relax. This
is the cycle that happens automatically when your cells are working the way
they should.

Now imagine standing in front of that terrifying crowd all day, every
day, with nowhere to go. This is how Mark felt. Because of a "perfect storm"
of stressors, his cells were stuck in the "on" stress response position, and he
was in a tailspin of worry, anxiety, and sleepless fight-or-flight mode. Day
after day with no relief caused significant wear and tear on Mark's body,
and he was feeling it.

Cue the entrance of Mark's signal-enhancing drink. Vitamin C concen-
trates in the adrenal glands, where it plays two roles. Referred to as an anti-
stress vitamin, vitamin C helped regulate the release of stress hormones. It
also readily donated electrons to power up his cells and help their recovery.
The sodium and potassium then teamed up to manage the flow of those
healing electrons in and out of his cells. Matt's simple homemade drink
combined these three important vitamins and minerals, and this combination allowed his cells and entire body to return to a balanced state. Over
the course of a few months, Mark turned off his "fight-or-flight switch" and
found blessed relief from his anxiety and insomnia.

Mark doesn't work in health care. In fact, Mark runs a bike repair shop.
He has long hair and an impressive handlebar mustache that ends in two
shaggy sprays well below his chin. But after medications failed to solve his
problems, he figured out how his cells worked and found his own way back
to wellness using a combination of science, research, and remedies he could
make at home. Mark spent many sleepless nights, a lot of time, and tons of

energy figuring all of it out on his own, but you don't have to. *Living Well with Dr. Michelle* will teach you simple, practical ways to improve your cells' signaling and communication so you can turn up your energy long before you are unwell.

Signs That Your Cells Aren't Well

You know when to charge your cell phone from the little low-battery display at the top of the screen. Your body has similar indicators that tell you when your cellular batteries are low and need to be charged:

1. **Low Physical Energy:** First, you feel a drop in energy physically. Fatigue, muscle weakness, or a general feeling of being weary are common signs you need to pay attention to.
2. **Brain Fog:** Next, your mind starts struggling to concentrate, your brain feels like it is slowing down, and you can't make decisions as easily as you normally could.
3. **Mood Swings:** Lastly, you start getting irritable, your mood swings widely, and you feel drained emotionally.

Indicators of Low Energy

Physical—Fatigue, muscle weakness, overall weariness

Mental—Poor concentration, sluggish brain, decreased decision-making ability

Emotional—Irritability, mood swings, emotionally drained

None of these symptoms will be new to you. But you have probably never been told that they are all signs of the same condition: low cellular energy. Interestingly, you do read these energy indicators daily, groaning and complaining, "I am so drained!" "I have no energy!" and "I am so dead today!" What do you do when all indicators show that your energy levels are low?

Recharge by simply giving your cells the electrons they need to thrive.

You've probably had a head cold at one time or another. While you were sick, your body was fighting invading germs, doing its best to kick them out and rebuild after their rampage through your cells and systems. To fight the infection, your cells required more energy than they do on a normal day, and to rebuild new, healthy cells, they required even more. If your body can't get extra cellular energy, it can't—and won't—be able to recover.

Where does your body get the extra cellular energy that it needs? These electrons are sourced from the planet's Five Elements. Societies have known about the medicine found in the earth for centuries, and modern science is beginning to name and define these sources with modern terminology, too. In *Living Well with Dr. Michelle,* you will learn how to use the electrons you get from the Five Elements as real medicine.

This is what Kate, the therapist you met earlier in the chapter, needed. Kate's cells were battling two formidable enemies. First, she had an infection in her jaw. But in their depleted state, her immune cells were attacking indiscriminately, destroying both allies and enemies. Caught in the crossfire, Kate's own cells were being destroyed, leading to relentless diarrhea and her immune system attacking her body, otherwise known as an autoimmune disease. Additionally, Kate had numerous metal plates in her leg from a serious accident years earlier, which disrupted the electron flow in her body. This interference prevented her cells from communicating effectively, exacerbating the situation. Kate's energy reserves were completely drained, leaving her cells without the electrons needed to fight.

Like Mark, Kate found the answers she needed by asking the right questions about what was happening to her cells: How did the infection affect her cells? What were the metal plates doing to her cells? Why had her cells become so depleted of energy in the first place? And most importantly, what did she need to do to help her cells and her body heal and repair themselves?

Kate started by having the infection in her jaw cleaned out, then diligently supported her healing cells by flooding her body with electrons. Some of those electrons came from the earth: Kate walked, sat, worked, and played as much as she could outside on the actual soil. Plants gather electrons from the sun, and Kate took those electrons in through simple but carefully planned plant-rich meals. Those foods also contained vitamins, minerals, and water, which improved her cellular communication and transportation systems, sending the electrons to where they were needed most. Additionally, Kate's own cells created more energy when she practiced deep breathing exercises every evening, consciously giving them more oxygen for fuel. To recap, Kate restored her cells to health by providing them with electrons, vitamins, minerals, water, and oxygen.

After three months of applying the simple healing methods that you're learning here in *Living Well with Dr. Michelle*, Kate started to feel and look like herself again. Her curly brown hair began growing back; she regained ten pounds of weight; and she was able to go back to work part-time in her practice. Kate was returning to health.

While the details of your health challenges will likely be different than Kate's, the steps you will take to return to wellness will be very similar.

Keyhole Concepts

For centuries, innovative gardeners have been planting "keyhole" gardens. This type of garden is a raised circular bed with a small section cut out of the middle, resembling a keyhole, which holds a composting basket. You fill the basket with kitchen scraps and yard waste, which decomposes and nourishes the soil. You then add layers of soil and compost around the basket, giving your vegetables or flowers the benefit of naturally rich soil to grow in. These gardens save space, enrich the soil naturally, are easy to access, and are largely self-sustaining.

I couldn't dream up a more appropriate metaphor to share at the end of each chapter than the Keyhole Concepts, modeled after this ingenious garden. The Keyhole Concepts will be just as concise, enriching, and easy to access as this garden, and they will guide you to self-sustaining wellness.

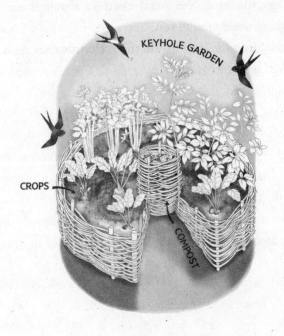

KEYHOLE GARDEN

CROPS

COMPOST

Chapter 1
Keyhole Concepts

+ Your body is doing the work and the healing, with support from doctors, pills, or bandages you are using.
+ You don't have to work to regain your health when you proactively give your cells what they need to stay well.
+ Cellular dysfunction and the resulting fallout is what we know as disease.
+ Disease care is doing something after the fact to help your cells and body return to correct function.
+ Wellness care is all about keeping the cells well in the first place.
+ Cell communication, called cell signaling, is essential for life.

+ Wellness comes from your cells and body communicating to keep you well.
+ The energy you need, the literal electrons that recharge cells, is found in the world around you.
+ The instructions for how to use those electrons are right here in *Living Well with Dr. Michelle*.

CHAPTER 2

Wellness Defined: Health Care Is More than Disease Care

When your cells aren't well, you aren't well. I learned this firsthand through years of illness. Though it was a difficult journey, understanding what was happening to my cells and my body changed my life. In this chapter, I'll share my personal journey back to health from mercury poisoning, a debilitating condition. You'll learn the importance of focusing on wellness care instead of disease care, and what the difference is between them. And you will finally understand what disease really is and isn't. Most importantly, you'll learn more about the fundamental roles your cells play in maintaining wellness and how you can best support their (and your) optimal health through the Cell Well model.

Michelle's Story

In 2010, after a decade and a half of studying and practicing dentistry and medicine so that I could keep others well, my own body was sick. As a young mom of four busy, growing children, I was stretched between a demanding business and a taxing home life. I had no energy and felt like I could barely keep my head above water. I couldn't sleep through the night or hold my dental instruments without pain and numbness in my hands and arms. My diet had been whittled down to a few "safe" foods that I could eat without stomach pain, and my once very sharp memory couldn't remember crucial details about patients and procedures. Something was very wrong, and my husband and I were worried.

I visited a plethora of doctors and had numerous blood tests, scopes, and X-rays, all to be told that the tests were inconclusive and that there was nothing wrong with me. The diagnosis I was given: stress. "Slow down," the doctors told me, "and things will get better." I left each visit with prescriptions for pills and procedures that the practitioners hoped would eliminate the symptoms. Nothing I was prescribed or recommended was an answer as to why my thirty-seven-year-old body seemed to be falling apart. For the first time in my life, I felt completely defeated. In desperation, I put my practice up for sale. I didn't want to leave dentistry, the career I had trained for and loved, but couldn't think of any other solution. At my wit's end, I decided to look for answers to my health problems outside of the medical establishment that I had been raised in and knew. I just couldn't give up hope that there was an answer, somewhere.

I started asking questions and talking to other dental practitioners who had struggled with health challenges. During one of these searching conversations, a new practitioner friend asked if I had considered mercury poisoning as a potential source of my problems. I laughed it off, explaining that I didn't have any "amalgam," or silver fillings, in my mouth. Years before, in a dental materials class, I had been taught those fillings contain mercury, but I had been quickly reassured that mercury in the fillings wasn't a problem for me or my patients. Now this in-the-trenches doctor was telling me differently. He said that regardless of what I had been taught, it would be wise to get tested. I knew that mercury was a highly toxic substance that can have serious health effects. Mercury primarily affects the nervous system, especially the brain, causing problems like shaking, memory issues, trouble focusing, and mood swings . . . all symptoms that I had been experiencing. So I decided to get tested. After all, what did I have to lose?

When my test results came back, I was floored. My mercury levels were so high they were off the charts. Finally, I had an answer, and it was simple. The mercury in those seemingly innocent fillings that I had been removing from my patients' teeth was poisoning me and my cells.[35] After learning about my toxic mercury levels, I swung between disbelief and anger that, as a dentist, I hadn't been warned about this inherent danger, and profound relief that I had an answer for what was causing my body's systems to fail.

Mercury in Dentistry?

How did this toxic metal come to be used in dentistry in the first place? The first mercury dental filling material was made in France in 1816 by a barber. In the 1800s, barbers weren't just cutting hair. They doubled as amateur doctors and dentists and were responsible for the development of a new type of tooth filling, called "amalgam." A barber mixed liquid mercury (that shiny stuff you see in old-fashioned glass-bulb thermometers) with shavings from silver coins and discovered that it formed a soft paste that could easily be packed into a hole in a tooth. After a few minutes, it would harden into a strong, long-lasting filling for cavities. Doctors, who also practiced dentistry in the 1800s, were concerned about the safety of these sturdy new fillings. They knew mercury was toxic and debated whether the benefits of this new filling material outweighed the potential risks of mercury exposure to patients and dental practitioners.

Doctors were familiar with the symptoms of mercury poisoning from treating hatmakers in England and France. In the eighteenth and nineteenth centuries, hat-making was a thriving industry in Europe, but the craft was lethal. That's because the process of creating felt hats involved mercury nitrate. This chemical was used to soften and mat animal (primarily rabbit) fur to create pliable and easier-to-shape felt for hats, a process known as "carroting" or "felting." Unfortunately for the hatters, that mercury exposure came with significant health risks. The symptoms appeared gradually and included tremors, headaches, mood swings, irritability, nervousness, mental health issues, speech problems, hallucinations, and, in severe cases, memory problems. Prolonged exposure to the toxic fumes and dust generated during the felting process led to mercury poisoning in hatters, and soon became known as "mad hatter's disease."[36]

Despite very legitimate safety concerns, the new mercury-containing filling material invented by European barbers was brought to the United States in 1830. It was an instant success. Inexpensive, easy to use, long-lasting, and fairly good at sealing the tooth, it became popular very quickly.

> As described by the FDA, "dental amalgam is a mixture of metals, consisting of liquid (elemental) mercury and a powdered alloy composed of silver, tin, and copper. Approximately half (50 percent) of dental amalgam is elemental mercury by weight."[37]

How Mercury Affects Cells

After learning about how mercury affected the hatmakers, I started to recognize similar symptoms in myself. Mercury can affect every cell in the body, and it leads to problems within all four of the Cell Well divisions of cell function:

Supply—Mercury sticks to enzymes, making it harder for the body to digest food, produce energy, and repair tissues.[38, 39, 40]

✦ **How it affected my cells' Supply functions:** After eating most foods, I had stomach pain, loose bowel movements, and low energy.

Support—Mercury causes stress in cells that harms your own proteins and DNA.[41] It can also lead to fertility problems, pregnancy issues like miscarriage and birth defects, and growth and development problems in children.[42, 43]

✦ **How it affected my cells' Support functions:** Sadly, I suffered from serious fertility problems for twenty years.

Secure—Mercury makes the cell walls less flexible and more leaky, causing imbalances inside the cell.[44] This can increase the risk of inflammation, heart attacks and strokes.[45]

+ **How it affected my Secure functions:** Mercury increased inflammation and swelling in my arms and hands, causing painful numbness that interfered with my ability to hold my dental instruments.

Signal—Mercury can enter cells in the brain, negatively affecting memory and movement. It can also cause cells to get confused in their signaling, leading to an early death for some.[46]

+ **How it affected my Signal functions:** I suffered from a failing memory and severe brain fog.

Wellness Instead of Disease Care

After I discovered my health problems stemmed from mercury poisoning, my life was consumed with disease care for more than five years. First, I had to get the mercury out, so I used a never-ending lineup of products that worked to pull the mercury from my organs. I felt like I had the flu for months on end as these medicines cleaned up my cells. After my cells were clean, I had to flood them with nutrients and antioxidants like vitamin C, vitamin E, and selenium to repair the damage. This is the perfect example of what I call "disease care"—treatment that is focused on specific symptoms and health problems someone already has. I am so grateful for the treatments that literally saved my life and career, but they were treating a disease, not helping me stay well.

If I'd known then what I do now, I would have worked to prevent the distress, illness, and disease my cells and I experienced. To put it simply, I didn't have to get sick. And other dental practitioners and patients don't have to either. If a dental school instructor, a colleague, or even a textbook had explained the risks of mercury to me, I could have taken the necessary proactive steps to protect my body and cells.

This is the foundation of wellness: taking the steps to proactively protect, support, build, and maintain your cells so you stay well and avoid disease. Wellness is based on understanding how each choice you make influences every cell. When you prevent illnesses and diseases before they occur, you'll extend both your lifespan and your healthspan.

Wellness

Focus: Wellness focuses on preventive measures and lifestyle interventions that promote and maintain overall cell and body health.

Approach: Wellness is about making proactive, informed, conscious choices about what you do and don't eat and drink, how you exercise and use your body, and how you can live a healthy lifestyle (for example, by not smoking).

Disease Care

Focus: Disease care, also known as sick care or medical care, primarily focuses on diagnosing and treating specific illnesses, injuries, or medical conditions.

Approach: Disease care happens after symptoms or diseases have already begun affecting health.

Modern medicine has largely become focused on disease and disease care, but this focus is negatively affecting wellness globally. Chronic diseases are among the leading causes of death in the United States, with heart disease and cancer alone accounting for around 38 percent of all deaths.[47] Nearly 122 million Americans (48 percent of adults) have cardiovascular disease,[48] and the number of people with arthritis is expected to increase to 67 million by 2030.[49] Over the past twenty years, the number of adults with diabetes has more than doubled,[50] and the latest report from the World Health Organization predicts that there will be more than thirty-five million new cases of cancer by 2050.[51]

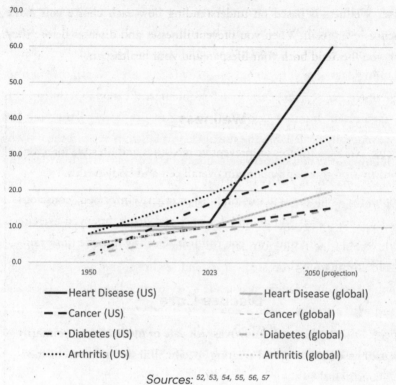

Trends in Chronic Diseases in the US and Globally
(1950, 2023, 2050)

Sources: [52, 53, 54, 55, 56, 57]

With all the new medical innovations in recent years, why are the numbers still going in the wrong direction? The answer is simple. We're focusing on the wrong thing: disease, not wellness.

The story of a dynamic mother-daughter duo, Sharon and Maggie, vividly demonstrates the difference between a disease approach versus a wellness approach. Sharon began struggling with joint pain even as a young adult and had reason to worry she would become like her father with thick, sore, and swollen arthritic joints. She watched her own hands for signs, knowing the arthritis was getting worse when her rings no longer slid easily over her fingers. Her knees began to ache, making walking a painful chore. Desperate for relief, Sharon visited her doctor to get cortisone injections in her knees. The injections did provide temporary relief, but each time the pain returned, it was more intense. The doctor warned that eventually, a total knee replacement would be necessary. Determined to postpone the surgery, Sharon even tried stem cell injections in her knees, but her knees were too far gone. When the pain became unbearable, she had her knees replaced, one at a time. The pain medication after surgery made her violently ill, causing days of relentless vomiting. To make matters worse, the anesthesia disrupted her heart rhythm, which required medication to stabilize. This new medication induced insomnia, adding to her misery. Although her knees eventually healed, Sharon's struggle was far from over. In the months that followed, she battled persistent insomnia and heart irregularities. The ordeal left Sharon very wary of further surgery.

Witnessing her mother's struggle, Sharon's daughter Maggie was determined to take a different path. She embraced a proactive approach to her health. She started taking turmeric supplements, drinking turmeric ginger tea, and eliminating processed sugars and seed oils from her diet to combat inflammation. Maggie also made sure to stretch before exercise and worked with a trainer to learn how to hike and work out without putting undue stress on her knees. Whenever she felt a twinge of pain, she applied arnica and magnesium cream, supplemented with Boswellia and cat's-claw to reduce inflammation.

Now age fifty-one, Maggie runs three times a week with no knee pain. Occasionally, the knuckles in her hands swell, but she can usually trace it back to a rare indulgence in sugar. With these lifestyle changes, Maggie feels confident that she will avoid the same arthritis story as her mother and grandfather. She understood that to be well you need to take this kind of proactive action to prevent illness.

How does this work? When you experience a symptom of disease, your next steps should be:

✦ Pay attention to and interpret early warning symptoms so that you can work to prevent more serious diseases from developing.
✦ Add power and energy to every cell by giving each of them the nutrients that they need to reverse symptoms and return your body to health.

Thankfully, I got a second chance to help myself be well. My journey, which was similar to the journey of thousands of my patients, progressed through the following stages:

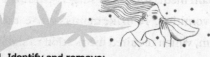

1. Identify and remove:
Determining that my problem was mercury poisoning wasn't easy, and figuring out what the solution was wasn't easy either.
My body couldnt flush the mercury out while I continued to remove mercury fillings for my patients.
If I wanted to continue to practice dentistry, I realized I would have to find a way to remove those fillings without getting more mercury exposure.

2. Create a healing environment:
After a deep-dive internet search, I found an organization that had already created safe mercury removal protocols. I made some essential changes to my office and procedures, purchased large mercury removal vacuums, and ordered special mercury filtration masks and impermeable clinical jackets for me and my team.

3. Provide the cells with healing energy:
My physical strength, stamina and vitality were at an all-time low, and mentally I was depressed. I had to find a way to provide my cells with what they needed to repair and heal so my body could do the same.
What did they need? Energy. Not the kind of energy you may complain about running out of after an exhausting day at work at 5PM on a workday. I'm talking about electrons and cellular energy.

If you are wondering how cells obtain these energy-giving electrons, the answer is simple: your cells get electrons from the food you eat, the water you drink, the air you breathe, and the earth you stand on. Once I learned about those natural elements, and how to get energy from them, I was able to help my body accelerate its own healing.

The key here is that my cells did the actual work: they released the mercury they were holding, helped remove it from my body, and finally repaired and rebuilt what had been damaged. I learned firsthand that your body knows what to do if you give your cells what they need to do it.

As I explain mercury and detoxing, cells and energy, you might be questioning the validity of this approach to wellness. You might even be giving me a teenage eye roll or two. I have dealt with a lot of questioning inside and outside my profession as I have shared my story and what I've learned over the last fifteen years. Other dentists have even challenged the idea that amalgam fillings can release enough mercury to make someone sick, how common the problem really is, and if it's being diagnosed accurately. Some believe my symptoms might have been caused by other health issues. When it comes to the natural detox methods I used, skeptics are doubtful about their effectiveness and safety.

These kinds of questions might be coming up for you at this point or later in the book as well. Questioning is a healthy way to evaluate new concepts. "Healthy skepticism" is powerful because it allows each one of us to critically assess information, leading to a deeper understanding of these complex subjects. In science, skepticism is essential for testing hypotheses and theories, and in fact, it drives the scientific method, ensuring that conclusions are based on rigorous evidence and reproducible results. My own deep questions started my health journey, science validated and confirmed what I learned, and thousands of patients and their stories reassured me that I am on the right track. This is the way we all learn, and this kind of questioning allows us to maintain an open mind and learn together.

So keep your mind open, ask, wonder, and ponder as you continue with me on this journey. We are just getting started!

The Details of Detoxing

Here's what I did, daily, to give my cells what they needed to heal. As you will see, my "medicine" was simply the electrons and energy that are contained in naturally occurring elements.

✳ ☆ Mercury Detox Steps ☆ ✳

Take Toxins Out

Drink: At least two quarts of clean, chlorine- and fluoride-free water per day to help both kidney and intestinal excretion. Water filtration information in chapter nine

Kidneys are the most important elimination route for the elemental mercury found in amalgam fillings.

Eat: Ensure that your diet is high in fiber with foods like berries, avocados, carrots, broccoli, black beans and sweet potatoes.
Supplement with magnesium in the evening.
Try Savory Crockpot Lentil Stew and Six-Can Chili (see Appendix 1 of this book for recipes).

Heavy metals are removed from cells, excreted through the liver, and dumped into the intestines. If your bowels are not working well, those toxins can be re-absorbed again.

Sweat: Break a sweat every day and shower it off. Exercise, infrared saunas, and mineral baths can all be used to promote the elimination of toxins through the skin.

Sweating is a great way to remove toxins from the body. See detox bath instructions.

✳ Put Nutrients In

Vitamins: Start the day with a smoothie including detoxing greens and fruit with vitamin C.
Try Morning Detox Smoothie.

Vitamin C is a potent antioxidant that helps stop the damage mercury can cause in cells.

Minerals: Take a liquid mineral supplement mixed with two cups of water, three times a day. Add a handful of Brazil nuts, sunflower seeds, or pumpkin seeds for the selenium and zinc.

Together, minerals and enzymes support your body processes by binding to toxins and removing them from from your cells.

Sulfur: Take or eat a sulfur-containing supplement called liposomal glutathione, or sulfur-containing foods like eggs, garlic, onions, broccoli, and cauliflower daily.
Try Oven Roasted Broccoli.

Mercury binds tightly to sulfur, and your body uses a sulfur molecule called glutathione to remove heavy metals from the body.

Sources: 58, 59, 60, 61, 62, 63, 64

Mistaken Definitions

Through my long and winding journey to return to wellness, I learned something profound yet simple: cells are much like people. They get tired, run-down, backed-up, sick, inflamed, and slow. They send signals when they aren't well that we call symptoms: digestive upset, headache, joint soreness, fatigue, anxiety, weight gain, weight loss, and more.

In the modern medical model, these symptoms are grouped together and called "disease." For example, when I was sick, I had symptoms such as digestive pain, constipation, and negative reactions to certain foods, and I felt bad after nearly every meal. My modern medical diagnosis was "irritable bowel syndrome" (IBS), a disease. I was given a referral to an allergist, had scopes to check out the insides of my digestive tract, was prescribed an acid-reducing pill, and was told this was something I would have to live with for the rest of my life.

All these recommendations and prescriptions were aimed at quieting the symptoms—the signals—my cells were sending. None of the diagnoses or treatments had anything to do with helping my cells return to health or be well. They were all reactive, with no options for treating what really ailed me and my cells. According to studies, IBS affects about 10–20 percent of the population.[65] I had become a statistic. But I knew there had to be a better way.

The fact is, people who are well do not need to manage symptoms, or even manage their health; they manage their cells.

By the time you have one of these "diseases," your cells are long past healthy, and you are probably very sick. There are many earlier signs and indicators—cell signals—that you will learn to pay attention to and respond to. Being misdiagnosed with irritable bowel syndrome when I really had mercury poisoning led to a difficult ten years for me, but from those challenges I learned firsthand what cells require to be well. And the Cell Well model of medicine was born. Now it will help you and countless other people be well, too.

Again, the premise of the Cell Well model is simple: when you help one cell be well, you help all your cells be well.

As you have learned, cells are tiny, microscopic units that are essential to life. They are often referred to as the "building blocks of life" because they are the basic structural and functional units of all living things. Here are some key things that your cells do for you:

Key Functions of Cells

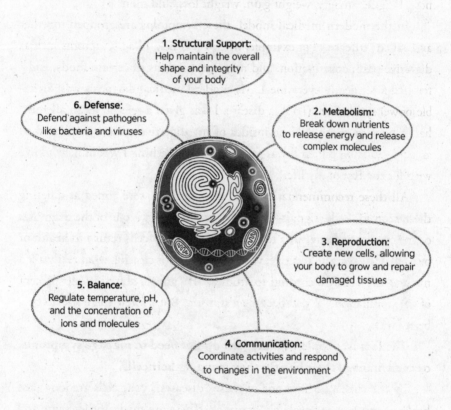

1. Structural Support: Help maintain the overall shape and integrity of your body

6. Defense: Defend against pathogens like bacteria and viruses

2. Metabolism: Break down nutrients to release energy and release complex molecules

3. Reproduction: Create new cells, allowing your body to grow and repair damaged tissues

5. Balance: Regulate temperature, pH, and the concentration of ions and molecules

4. Communication: Coordinate activities and respond to changes in the environment

Overall, cells are incredibly versatile and dynamic entities that work together to keep living organisms, including you, alive and functioning properly. Without cells, life as you know it would not be possible.

The Living Well Cell

A Living Well Cell is a cell that is functioning optimally and working effectively in an ecosystem with other cells. Although there are many specific types of cells in your body—including muscle cells that contract, nerve cells that transmit electrical signals, and blood cells that circulate nutrients—there are some essential things that all cells require, twenty-four seven, to operate. In the cellular ecosystem, these essential functions are grouped into four main divisions, which were introduced in chapter 1. To keep a cell well, you need to provide what the cell needs for all these functions.

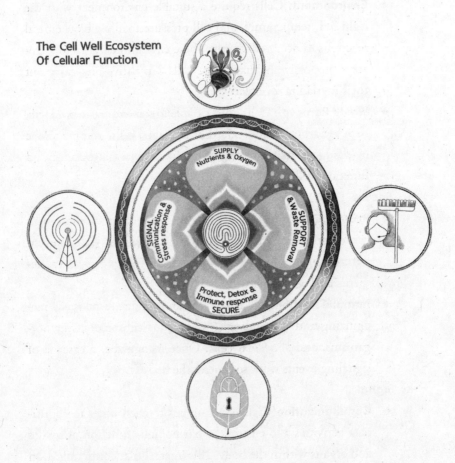

The Cell Well Ecosystem
Of Cellular Function

1. **Supply**
   + **Nutrients:** All cells require a constant supply of nutrients to carry out their metabolic processes and energy production. These nutrients include carbohydrates, proteins, fats, vitamins, and minerals.

✦ **Oxygen:** Cells also need oxygen to support cellular respiration, the process by which they generate energy from nutrients. Oxygen is essential to produce adenosine triphosphate, or ATP, the molecule that serves as the primary energy source for cellular activities.

2. **Support**

✦ **Environment:** Cells require a suitable environment with the right pH, temperature, and cell pressure to allow biochemical reactions to occur efficiently. These environmental factors create a supportive habitat where cells can thrive and carry out their myriad tasks effectively.

✦ **Waste Removal:** Cells must be able to remove waste products, such as carbon dioxide, dead or damaged cells, and metabolic by-products, to allow cells to maintain internal balance and function well.

3. **Secure**

✦ **Protect/Detox:** Cells must be able to select which substances can enter or exit the cell. The cell's barriers or walls prevent harmful agents from entering and actively pump toxic elements back out as needed.

✦ **Immune Response:** Cells mount an immune response by recognizing and responding to dangerous substances, microorganisms, and abnormal cells. Once recognized, a cascade of signaling events work to protect the body.

4. **Signal**

✦ **Communication:** Cells send signals to each other to coordinate activities and ensure the harmonious function of tissues and organs within the body. This intercellular communication occurs through a variety of signaling mechanisms.

✦ **Stress Response:** Cells can respond to various forms of stress, including environmental changes, pathogens, physiological challenges, and cellular damage. These stress responses are crucial for promoting survival and ensuring proper function.

The Cell Well model is all about proactively providing your cells with everything they need to be well—the opposite of modern medicine's reactive disease care model. What I learned from being my own "patient zero" was that I had to help my cells and focus, every day, on giving my cells exactly what they needed to heal. The journey I took wasn't easy at the time, and honestly, it still isn't. Shifting my focus to wellness was challenging, but it was worth it. My body is living well again, and I feel it in every cell. You can, and will, too.

Chapter 2
Keyhole Concepts

- ✦ Wellness refers to all the proactive measures you can use to promote and maintain your overall health and prevent disease. Disease care focuses on diagnosing and treating specific health conditions you already have.
- ✦ Modern medicine has largely become focused on disease, and this focus is negatively affecting wellness globally.
- ✦ Cells get electrons from the food you eat, the water you drink, the air you breathe, and the earth you stand on.
- ✦ Cells can get tired, run-down, backed-up, sick, inflamed, and slow. When that happens, cells send signals that you experience as symptoms: digestive upset, headache, joint soreness, fatigue, anxiety, weight gain or weight loss, and more. These symptoms warn you that things aren't right in your cells.
- ✦ Truly healthy people do not need to manage symptoms, or even manage their health; they manage their cells.
- ✦ When you help one cell be well, you help all your cells be well.
- ✦ Wellness care is based on understanding how each choice you make influences every cell. The goal of wellness care is to prevent illnesses and diseases before they occur, extending both lifespan and healthspan.

CHAPTER 3

Wellness Challenged: Your Cells Are Up to the Challenge

Let's face it, we live in a toxic world. Toxins made me sick, and they have the potential to make you sick, too. Toxins are present in the air you breathe, even if you can't see them. Microscopic contaminants make their way into your cells through the water you drink. Foods can carry harmful hitchhikers in many forms, such as bacteria, mold, pesticides, dangerous fats, dyes, and additives. You may unknowingly apply nice-smelling poisons in the form of shampoo and perfumes, and your cell phone and Wi-Fi connection constantly expose you to invisible electronic irritants.

How do you and your cells survive this toxic onslaught?

Furthermore, your parents and grandparents may have suffered from heart conditions, diabetes, high blood pressure, or various forms of cancer. Maybe you feel that you will now inevitably suffer from those diseases as well because you've inherited their genes.

Fortunately, your cells and body are adept at adapting and changing to meet the challenges they encounter—whether environmental or genetic. You just need to know what steps to take to support them. You aren't a prisoner of your circumstances or your DNA!

Nature or Nurture?

Is wellness predetermined by the genes you were born with? Do your cells and body follow a rigid, unalterable genetic code? Are your health and future predestined because of your DNA?

Nature versus nurture . . . this question has been asked in scientific and philosophical circles for hundreds of years, but a tiny boy named Eric brought the question to life for me. From the moment he took his first breath as a teeny tiny preemie, Eric was challenged. Many of his organs and cellular systems weren't fully formed before he was born. After four and a half months in the neonatal intensive care unit, Eric was sent home with a feeding tube, oxygen, and sleep apnea monitor.

All of Eric's typical childhood milestones were delayed. He finally smiled, rolled over, and learned to eat on his own well enough to have his feeding tube removed by his first birthday. By his second birthday, Eric could make it through the day without receiving extra oxygen, and he was starting to be mobile, scooting across the floor on his bottom. At two and a half, Eric's family was thrilled when he started walking and pulling his little red wagon around, but they could also no longer ignore the signs of other serious developmental delays. Eric was completely nonverbal and didn't seem to understand words or what they meant. At thirty-two months old, testing found Eric to be functioning at an eight-month-old level. And there were other issues, too, including a mouth so small that even tiny baby teeth had nowhere to fit.

Eric's family was stumped. How had his development gotten so off-track? And why? They wondered if his cells were genetically programmed to perform this way, or whether they were influenced by the challenges of his premature birth, nutritional deficiencies, and low oxygen.

In the last fifty years, a vast amount of information about cells has been amassed. However, scientists still have a lot to learn about how the genes in even the simplest bacteria provide instructions for all its cells to grow, let alone how they guide the growth of a human with around thirty thousand genes and cells numbering in the trillions. Scientists believe they will one day fully map out all our inner workings, like studying a complex machine.

But others, myself included, think that this is looking at cells and the way they function through the wrong lens. People aren't computers to be coded or car engines to be tuned. There are no static or absolute answers when working with living, breathing, changeable organisms like the human body and its cells. To get a better understanding of what I mean, let's turn to nature and look at some living things you are familiar with, to simplify and explain cells and how they function.

People, and Their Cells, Aren't Machines

During the Scientific Revolution in the sixteenth and seventeenth centuries, scientists viewed cells as intricate machines with a design, structure, and operation that followed predictable laws. Machine analogies and metaphors such as "motor," "engine," and "well-oiled machine" became a popular way to describe living cells and are still in use today.[66] Following the Second World War, these analogies expanded as new concepts in computer science captured the imagination of biologists. Computers (which are also machines) have "software" and "hardware," and those concepts were applied to describe how cells work as well.

This idea of the "cell as a machine" influenced the birth of modern molecular biology, in which the cells and body are seen as a system of genetic coding (software) and molecular components (hardware). Today, many people still believe that cells operate in a fixed, mechanical way according to a genetic program encoded in DNA. In this model, this DNA "instruction manual" directs the formation of cellular parts and pieces that are then assembled into molecular machines. These machines perform pre-programmed tasks, and when things go wrong, the DNA coding or instructions are to blame.

But unlike humans, machines don't live or breathe or remember or change. Science and those trying to explain it have leaned heavily on machine analogies to explain the body, but this has set medical practitioners up for frustration. Bodies and their systems, which are organic in nature, can't be expected to operate like machines. Unforeseen and sometimes unexplainable things happen in bodies and cells, including Eric's perplexing growth challenges. As a dentist, I was stumped by his small mouth with inadequate room for his teeth and tongue. If the programming for his mouth size came from his inherited DNA "software," why were his mother's and father's mouths normal-sized? If his cells contained genetic instructions to grow lungs and other organs and vessels, why did Eric have to have a string of surgeries before age one to move organs and vessels to the correct place in his little body? As I continued to question what had led to Eric's growth challenges, it became clear there was something missing in my understanding about what can and can't affect cells and the way they develop and work.

The "cells are like machines" model proposes that cells have been pre-programmed and will function in one way only based on that programming. This classic cell model that you probably learned in high school is being increasingly questioned. Cells are not lifeless combinations of wires and circuits. Cells are full to overflowing with billions of colliding, interacting molecules that are in constant motion. Unlike a computer, with its predictable operations and precise components, cells are unpredictable, and their behavior depends on their environment. Macrophages, the versatile superheroes of the immune system, are a great example of this. They adapt their behavior based on what the body needs. When invaders such as bacteria or viruses strike, these cells become fierce warriors fighting to protect our bodies. They engulf and destroy the pathogens in a process not unlike Pac-Man gobbling up dots. However, in an environment with chronic inflammation, macrophages switch gears from fighters to healers. They start cleaning up the damaged cells and tissue, repairing damages and even forming scar tissue if necessary, much like a construction crew fixing up a building after a storm. This dual nature allows macrophages to be incredibly effective whether they're battling infections or helping the body heal.[67]

Perhaps the only way to really understand all that is happening in a cell would be to shrink a scientist with a video camera down to a very small size and send them into a cell to record the action.[68] In the absence of a miniature scientist with reality-show footage, I've put together what I've learned about cells into a new, more human, less mechanical model that better explains how they really work.

Like Your Home, Cells are Changeable

Growing up, I would occasionally eat dinner with my best friend, either at her house or mine. When eating at her house, we knew exactly what we would eat. Monday was hamburger patties covered in tangy tomato sauce. Tuesday was tacos with greasy, delicious tortillas straight out of the frying pan. Every day had a menu that was followed predictably. Meals at my home were the opposite. My mom grew up eating a similar menu to what was found at my friend's home, and she wanted something different for her family. At my house, we ate salmon before anyone knew it was good for us and tried "exotic" delicacies like Greek olives and asparagus. You never knew what would fill your belly until you were sitting at the table—it was a delicious roll of the dice every evening. Neither dinner table was right or wrong; they were just different. My friend's mother followed the same recipes every week with precision, but my mother followed her whims and appetite.

Like family dinner tables, cells can be predictable sometimes and unpredictable other times, depending on the environment. This doesn't fit well in the classic "cells as machines" model where everything is predictable, and DNA is responsible for any problem. Using this model to explain Eric's situation, scientists might say his developmental path was programmed and inevitable; once set, it was as unchangeable as a recipe in a cookbook. In this model, the only way to change the way a cell acts is to make changes to the genes or DNA. But when my mother wanted to change up our meal for the night, she didn't have to buy a new recipe book altogether, she simply turned to another page in the recipe book she already owned. It's the same with your cells and body.

You don't have to change your DNA to change the way your cells and body behave.

To really understand this, you have to throw out the machine understanding of cell function. New research shows that DNA doesn't program one set recipe, an immutable set of instructions for how your cells should function; DNA simply tells your body how to make new cells. The operations and instructions for those new cells are transmitted from cell to cell through electrical signals.[69] And those instructions are changeable based on the cell and the environment the cell lives in.

To see this in action, let's take a journey through the body. If you did join that miniature scientist and were to shrink down to the size of a cell, how would you know which organ neighborhood you were traveling through? Looking around, you would see there are around two hundred different types of cells your DNA can tell your body to make. While they are all similar in some ways, many have very different shapes, sizes, and functions. Let's look more closely at two different types: brain cells and blood cells.

The brain is like the operations manager of your body. It runs the receiving department, processing information from the environment and instructing the other organs what to do with that information. When it starts to rain outside, your brain processes this environmental change and tells your muscles to contract so they can move your body toward shelter. To send those instructions, the brain cells need to transmit electric or chemical signals to the cells in the muscles in your legs and feet. Those signals must travel a long way to get from your brain to your feet. For this to happen quickly and efficiently, your DNA has a recipe for a specific type of nerve cell with long branches off the main cell body—which can reach a length of up to three feet![70] This unique structure enables the nerve cells to pass signaled instructions from the brain to muscles as far away as your pinky toe very quickly.

These cells look very different than blood cells. Red blood cells move oxygen from your lungs to other organs so that those organs can keep producing energy. These tiny cells can move around your entire body in just twenty seconds![71] They are shaped differently than nerve cells because they serve a different function. Long, lanky nerve cells can't move this quickly and would get tangled up in a system like the bloodstream. To help them get where they need to go, blood cells are small and have a flattened disk shape, similar to a doughnut without the hole. This shape gives them a lot of surface area for oxygen to bind to.

The answer to which neighborhood you are in can be found in the cells in that neighborhood. The structure and function of cells differ depending on the organs in which they are found. But here is the more important question: if each cell in your body has a set of the same exact DNA (which it does), how does your body know how and when to make one cell type or another? Cells are smart! They use a very sophisticated control mechanism to make sure that only the correct genes (pieces of information on the DNA) are used, and the genes that are used determine the cell type that is made.

Compare this to the process used to bake different kinds of muffins. Some ingredients, including eggs, flour, and milk, are the same in every muffin, but different muffins require special additional ingredients, like apples, cinnamon, or blueberries depending on the muffin flavor you

Different Cellular Recipes Instruct Different Cell Types

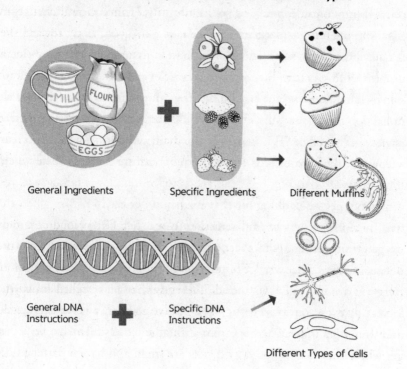

General Ingredients   Specific Ingredients   Different Muffins

General DNA Instructions   Specific DNA Instructions

Different Types of Cells

want. Your cells' recipe book, the DNA, is housed in the nucleus or cellular library found inside every cell. This book contains recipes for making all the necessary cell types. Depending on what they need, neighborhoods send signals instructing new cells to choose one recipe over another. Once the cell knows what it needs to become or do, it will now read only the portion of the DNA that is applicable to those processes. This is all done without physically changing any of the cell's DNA or parts.[72]

We Can Help Our Bodies and Cells during Challenges

This ability to read individual portions of the DNA, or recipes, means that you can greatly change the way a cell, an organ, and even your whole body behaves by giving it signals to read a new recipe. Of course, toxins and other environmental contaminants can also send signals that influence your cells' recipe choices in a negative way. This is an everyday challenge for all of your cells—but one you can defend yourself against. Think about it like taking a walk in the rain. Without an umbrella, you are going to get soaking wet. It's inevitable. But with a little planning and forethought, you can bring an umbrella and stay dry. The food you choose to eat, the water you drink, the soil you stand on, and the air you breathe can give you a literal umbrella of protection from the toxins, environmental contaminants, and genetic challenges that you face. This is nature's medicine, and learning how to use it properly will help your cells and your body both stay well and heal quickly if necessary.

Many people, looking for that medicine, retreat to nature when they need to think or pray or find direction in life. I call it "sitting on a rock." There is something about the earth and her beautiful places that draws people in. Have you ever "communed with" the trees or the waves or the hills you are visiting? This sounds New Agey, but it's backed by science. Changing even your physical environment can significantly alter your cellular function, improving both your mental and physical wellness. "Forest bathing," or using your senses to experience the forest, can lead to remarkable changes in your body. When you walk through a forest, breathe in fresh air, and surround yourself with trees, your body produces less cortisol (a stress hormone) and your stress levels drop.[73] Trees also release natural oils called phytoncides into the air which boost your immune system, cuing your body to increase the activity of cells crucial in fighting off infections and even cancer.[74] Being in nature even boosts serotonin levels in your brain, improving your mood and thinking ability, making you feel happier and more focused.[75]

Incorporating nature into your routine can fundamentally change how your cells function. Start by visiting a local park or nature reserve once a week, walking slowly to fully engage your senses with the environment. Sit quietly under a tree or near a stream, practicing mindfulness by focusing on the sights, sounds, and smells around you. Add physical activities like yoga or tai chi to further enhance the benefits. This environmental change significantly impacts you and your cells, and you can literally feel it.

How do your cells know you are in a forest or looking at a beautiful flower? Your eyes, ears, nose, and skin send information to your brain, immune system, and other systems at lightning speed. Nature gives us examples of how this works. Whether it's a sunflower, a hive full of bees, or a coral reef, everything in nature has a system that can be used for communication.[76] As you walk in the forest, or your own neighborhood, you might see tree trunks, branches, and leaves, but to understand how trees communicate with each other, you need to look beneath the soil to learn about their hidden communication networks. Trees live in cooperative, interdependent societies, maintained and supported by shared information. They are connected to each other through underground fungal networks and through chemical messages they send back and forth. They share water, nutrients, distress signals about drought and disease, and even warn about animal or insect attacks. Other connected trees change their behavior when they receive these messages. Researchers jokingly call this the "wood-wide web"![77]

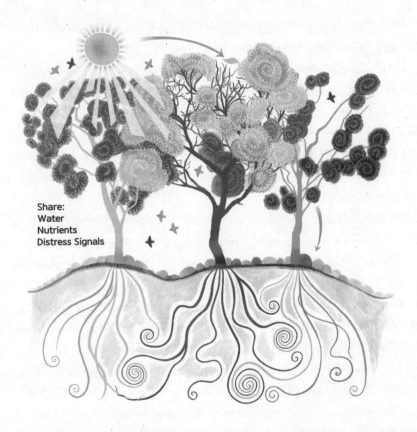

Share:
Water
Nutrients
Distress Signals

Across Africa and the Middle East, the umbrella thorn acacia tree thrives because of this amazing tree communication system. It grows in sand dunes and rocky grounds, surviving in areas with annual rainfall as low as four inches, temperatures soaring to over 122 degrees Fahrenheit during the day, and freezing temperatures at night. It grows up to seventy feet high with a spreading, flat-topped crown that gives it its name. With black bark, gnarled branches, and two types of prickly thorns, this tree is a testament to survival. It has adapted to its environment in startling ways, including growing a long, deep taproot that can extend up to 155 feet under the soil. This allows the tree to harvest the last drops of water that will help it pull through dry spells and droughts. The wide spread of its branches enables the tree to capture the greatest amount of sunlight with the smallest possible leaves. This minimizes water loss, and the spiky thorns deter animals from eating the leaves, flowers, and seeds.

The only animal able to tolerate the wide crowned acacia's thorns and get to the foliage is the gangly giraffe! But the tree's communication system has adapted to evade even these hungry animals. When a giraffe starts chewing the leaves of the acacia tree, the tree has a cellular defense recipe for how to respond. It signals its leaf cells to create bitter compounds called tannins that sicken and even kill giraffes. The injured tree then follows a second cellular recipe and sends out a distress signal to other neighboring trees by emitting ethylene gas. When the neighboring trees detect this gas, their leaf cells also create bitter tannins, deterring giraffes from feeding on their leaves.

Acacias aren't the only organisms that can change their cellular behavior based on their environment. In a humorous twist of nature, the giraffe's cells have changed along with the acacias. Wanting to avoid a bitter surprise, giraffes only browse on acacia trees that are upwind from other acacias, so the warning gas doesn't reach the neighboring trees ahead of them. If there is no wind, a giraffe simply walks further than the ethylene gas can travel before munching on another tree. Giraffes know that the trees can communicate with each other and have altered their own actions in response. Why do trees and giraffes communicate and warn and defend one another? The answer is survival. They are stronger and survive longer when they remember how to respond to challenges and share what they have learned with each other. Your cells have changed to survive, too.

Despite being bombarded by a diverse array of challenges, the DNA inside each human cell stores information on how to survive. My friend Macy experienced this firsthand when she decided to move to Cusco, Peru. Hearing it was a cultural mecca, she packed up her bags and took the long trek to her new home. As soon as she arrived, she noticed she couldn't quite catch her breath. The city is perched at the top of a mountain at more than eleven thousand feet of elevation. The air is "thinner" at this elevation, meaning each breath delivered less oxygen to Macy's cells, and she found herself breathing more heavily and feeling lightheaded. The locals were quick to explain that she was experiencing altitude sickness, and it could potentially be very dangerous. Questioning her decision to move, Macy followed their suggestions to take it easy for a few days, drink a lot of water, and avoid alcohol and caffeine. Thankfully, within a few weeks the problems with her breathing nearly disappeared. What happened? How did she get acclimated to the higher elevation and thinner air?

A growing body of research suggests that trauma in humans (from abuse, food insecurity, or thin air, among other things) makes a chemical mark on the DNA. Think of it like a note in the margins on the DNA recipe book, telling the cook to use a little more salt or bake the dish for five minutes longer than the recipe instructs. When that DNA is passed from parent to child, the notes are passed down as well. This note or mark doesn't change the actual recipe or DNA, but it changes the way the body reads the DNA. This note isn't a genetic change or mutation. It is something entirely different, called an "epigenetic" change.[78] Macy didn't change her DNA or grow new lung cells when she was struggling to get enough oxygen. Her lung cells, prompted by the low oxygen, read a little note on her DNA that had been passed down from an ancestor before her. This note signaled her body to make more red blood cells when they encountered low oxygen levels, which then carried more oxygen from her lungs to the rest of her cells.

We will continue to talk about this concept of notes and DNA recipes because it is key in the Cell Well model. Once you know how to update your cellular recipe books, you can change the way your cells and body work and infinitely increase your wellness.

Notes and DNA Recipes

The idea of epigenetic influence was pioneered by a British developmental biologist, Conrad Hal Waddington, whose ideas have reshaped the understanding of how organisms develop and evolve. In the 1950s, Waddington introduced the concept of an "epigenetic landscape" in an attempt to describe how genes interact with their environment during development. He used the analogy of a ball rolling down a hill to illustrate how development is influenced by both genetic and environmental factors. DNA programs the way the ball forms, but as the ball rolls down the hill, it bumps and bounces in and out of ridges and depressions of the landscape, eventually settling into one of many possible valleys at the bottom.

In Waddington's model, the ridges, depressions, and variations represent environmental factors such as diet, stress, and exposure to toxins. The final valley the ball ends up in depends largely on which of those factors the ball encounters on the way down the hill. Although Waddington's original concept of the epigenetic landscape has been refined and expanded upon over the years, its core idea, that development is the result of the ongoing interaction between genes and the environment, continues to be a guiding principle in modern biology.

In recent years, Dr. David Sinclair and his colleagues at Harvard Medical School have taken Waddington's work and expanded it to the study of aging. I'm at what I would consider to be the midpoint of my life, and I'm starting to see and feel some unwelcome signs of aging. My skin sags in areas it never did before, my knees and ankles crack, I have swollen fingers occasionally, and I certainly can't stray too far from the nearest restroom. While I've accepted these symptoms as part of growing older, research tells me that my aging cells are at increased risk for many diseases, including cancer, cardiovascular disease, diabetes, and brain and memory disorders.[79] This is a risk I would like to avoid. If cellular aging can be stopped or even reversed, it stands to reason that multiple age-related diseases could be delayed or eliminated.

Sinclair decided to focus on Waddington's "epigenome." As we've discussed, certain chemical compounds modify or mark the DNA or the cellular recipes in a way that tells the cell what to do, where to do it, and when to do it. There are three general types of marks or chemical tags that can change the epigenome. You can think of them like sticky notes, dog-eared pages, and handwritten recipe notes:

✦ **Sticky notes:** DNA methylation occurs when tiny groups of atoms, called methyl groups stick to specific spots on the cell's DNA. They tell the cell what to read and what to ignore.

- ✦ **Dog-eared pages:** Like bending the corner of your page down to mark your favorite recipe, histone modifications make genes easier or harder to find and read.
- ✦ **Handwritten notes:** Similar to the handwritten notes you might scribble at the top of a recipe, non-coding RNAs make tweaks to the DNA instructions without changing the recipe itself.

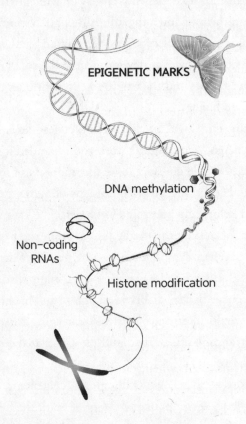

These epigenetic markings can be passed from cell to cell as they divide. That means that when a skin cell divides, the page to make that cell a skin cell is still dog-eared, and it forms another skin cell.[80]

Let's see how this works in living cells and bodies. Growing up, my family had a large garden where a colony of earthworms lived. On occasion, an unfortunate earthworm got in the way of a shovel while my brothers and I were digging weeds and would get cut in half by the sharp edge. We would watch in amazement as the two halves of the earthworm continued on their way as if nothing had happened, eventually growing back the rest of their bodies. The worm's DNA gave it the basic information, or recipe, telling it what to do when cut. But research shows that the worm's recipe book can be marked and read in another way, based on the worm's experiences or environment.

Planarians are a fascinating kind of flatworm that, when cut, will sometimes grow a head at each end instead of a tail. Scientists wanted to know if they could influence whether the worm grew a head or tail or one of each, essentially changing the way the planarian's DNA recipe is read.[81] They added a chemical called octanol to the water the worms were living in. Octanol interferes with the way cells send and receive electrical signals and makes an epigenetic mark on the worm's DNA. When the octanol-soaked worms were cut, 25 percent of them grew into a two-headed worm. The most important finding was that when researchers looked at the DNA of these two-headed worms, nothing had changed; it was identical to the DNA of the one-headed worms. The recipe was the same, but the markings changed the way it was read. Because of these studies and others, there is now conclusive evidence that cellular information is stored in two places: in the DNA, which is the recipe book for your cells, and in the epigenome, the permanent marks on the DNA that modify how it's read.

With this new information, Sinclair and his team concluded that cellular aging in humans occurs when your DNA recipe book loses its epigenetic marks—the critical instructions it needs to continue reading the recipes correctly. Dr. Sinclair further explains that we often consider the processes behind aging and age-related diseases as irreversible, but in some cases, existing cells are simply not functioning properly, and they can return to normal if you re-mark them. This represents a new way to approach medicine.[82] This suggests that the diseases that make us unwell, including chronic conditions like heart disease and neurodegenerative conditions like Alzheimer's, may be able to be prevented by marking and re-marking your body's cells and systems.

The Cell Well model aims to do just that.

How the Cell Well model can improve cell function through epigenetics

✦ **Supply** your cells with compounds that create "wellness marks" on your DNA. Folate and B vitamins like B6 and B12 are crucial for DNA methylation (sticky notes). Focus on a diet rich in leafy greens, legumes, and fish to get more of them.[83]

✦ **Support** your cells and DNA through physical activity. Activity induces beneficial histone modifications (dog-eared pages) that improve muscle function, metabolism, and brain health.[84]

✦ **Secure** your cells from cellular stress by adding green tea, berries, and turmeric to your diet to increase DNA methylation (sticky notes).[85]

✦ **Signal** your cells by decreasing stress. Chronic stress has been linked to the malfunction of non-coding RNAs (handwritten notes), especially the ones instructing your cells to avoid inflammation. Practice mindfulness and meditation to improve cellular and overall health.[86]

You and Your Cells Aren't Prisoners of Your DNA

Here's the best news! You aren't a prisoner of your DNA. You can stay well and heal from disease by making choices and taking actions that help your cells adapt to the challenges in their immediate environment and the world at large. That means that you will be able to thrive in nearly any situation.[87] What a relief to know that being well and staying well is not all about your DNA, and that disease is not inevitable. The study of epigenetics has given conclusive evidence that you can change your cells' information to preserve and improve your health.[88]

Eric's Epigenetic Journey to Health

Eric, the young boy with the small mouth and developmental delays, has cells and DNA full of recipes for growth and development, just like you. There are recipes for growing lungs, building vessels that connect the lungs to the heart, putting different organs in the right compartments, and running the power plants in each cell. However, because Eric was born fifteen weeks early, his genes didn't have time to follow the programming while he was developing in utero. His tiny, underdeveloped body was thrust into a hostile world of lights, sounds, and unwelcome air, food, and water. His lungs, vessels, and digestive system weren't ready for any of this. For four months, instead of being protected in his mother's body, his home was an incubator. While his body fought to catch up with this early entry into the world and his "ball" rolled down his developmental hill, it ran into some very significant rocks and bumps that nearly threw it off the hill completely. Because of these challenges, Eric's doctors and family weren't surprised when his development was delayed. He could have been forever impacted by severe communication, size, systemic health, and learning challenges, but luckily, epigenetic rebooting can happen at any age and stage. That is what had to happen for Eric's developmental "ball"; it had to be taken back to the top of the hill and allowed to follow a different course.

Eric was lucky because he had a family who devoted themselves completely to caring for his medical and developmental needs. Corrective surgeries, intensive speech, occupational and physical therapy, and plenty of nutritionally rich foods were all part of Eric's routine in the next few years. A well-meaning pediatrician's nurse told Eric's family that he would always have significant delays and impairments, but his family decided to see what making changes to his environment could do to help. Eric had a younger sister who modeled what a youngster his age should be doing. He followed her everywhere and copied everything she did. If she ate a new food, Eric would, too. If she babbled to herself while reading a book, Eric babbled right along with her. They slept in the same room, shared toys, and went to the park, church, and preschool together, activating "mirror neurons" in Eric's brain.

Mirror neurons are a type of neuron that fires both when someone performs an action themself or when they observe someone else performing the same action. They were first discovered in the 1990s by a team of researchers led by Giacomo Rizzolatti at the University of Parma in Italy. You might be familiar with mirror neurons in action from the phenomenon of contagious yawning: when you see someone else yawn, mirror neurons in your brain fire as if you were yawning yourself, leading you to involuntarily yawn in response. These cells are believed to be involved in a wide range of other social behaviors, such as imitation, learning through observation, and understanding the emotions of others.[89] These cells learn new instructions and then mirror what they see. This is reprogramming in action, and Eric was soon singing and dancing and reading books right along with his sister.

Reprogramming Eric's eating habits also helped Eric become healthier. With clear signs of malnutrition, Eric was always desperate for food. He would cry until his plate was full, then he would shove food into his mouth as quickly as he could until he made himself sick. Favoring quick-burning carbohydrates like crackers and French fries, Eric's nutritional needs weren't being met. His mom changed what filled Eric's plate, even if not having his favorite foods made him upset. She knew that foods with actual vitamins and minerals were what Eric really needed, and eventually Eric started favoring everything green, including broccoli, asparagus, peas, and beans, and self-selecting away from food that hampered his growth, like sugar and processed dairy products. Eric's little cheeks started plumping, he put on some weight, and he finally got well enough to undergo needed corrective surgeries.

Eric's challenged body had endured surgeries in the NICU that saved his life, but unbeknownst to anyone, one of those surgeries had failed. Eric's stomach had moved up through his diaphragm and into his chest cavity, crowding his heart and lungs. Extensive reconstructive surgery repositioned and repaired his digestive system. The work of doctors, therapists, and myself, a dentist, were important during Eric's next years. Due to his premature birth and the resulting damage to his digestive tract, he struggled to absorb essential nutrients during his early development. This malnutrition contributed to the underdevelopment of his upper jaw, leading to severe tooth crowding and an underbite, which further challenged his eating and speaking. Essentially, Eric's genetics and his epigenetics clashed. Eric's DNA contained programming for a proper-sized upper jaw, following the information in the genes from his mother and father. However, that information changed because of his premature birth and early lack of nutrients. A new nutrient-rich diet and continued medical care improved Eric's situation, but the jaw underdevelopment had already occurred. After multiple rounds of appliances and braces as his mouth and teeth grew, Eric now has a handsome smile with straight teeth, and he can chew and speak normally. This once little, malnourished, severely delayed child is now a fully functioning adult who graduated from school and is working in a job to help other kids who have struggles not unlike his own.

Addressing Skepticism and Misconceptions About Epigenetics and Cellular Health

It's natural for people to have questions or doubts about complex topics like epigenetics and cellular health. Here are some common misconceptions and clarifications for this complicated information:

1. **Misconception:** Epigenetics can change your DNA.
   + **Clarification:** Epigenetics does not change the DNA itself but influences how the information in the DNA or genes is expressed. Think of it like that dimmer switch for lights we talked about earlier—epigenetic changes can turn genes on or off or adjust their intensity without altering the underlying DNA.[90]
2. **Misconception:** Epigenetic changes are permanent.
   + **Clarification:** While some epigenetic changes can be long-lasting, especially those established early in life, others are reversible. The environment, lifestyle choices, and even therapeutic interventions can lead to changes in the epigenome, demonstrating its flexibility and adaptability.[91]

3. **Misconception:** Epigenetics is just a new buzzword with no real impact on health.
    + **Clarification:** Epigenetics is a well-established field of science that has been studied for decades. Research shows that epigenetic mechanisms play a crucial role in development, aging, and diseases such as cancer. Understanding epigenetics is essential for grasping how our bodies function and respond to various factors throughout life.[92]
4. **Misconception:** There's nothing you can do to change your genes.
    + **Clarification:** Your epigenome is dynamic and responsive to various factors like diet, exercise, stress, and exposure to toxins. By making healthy lifestyle choices, you can positively influence your epigenome, potentially improving your health and well-being.[93]

The Epigenome Learns from Its Experiences

How do these epigenetic marks change cells and DNA at the biochemical level? We have learned that each cell has a memory of all the signals or experiences it's encountered during its life. These experiences leave marks on the DNA, which guide the cell's behavior. This process starts as soon as an egg is fertilized. The fertilized egg contains DNA from both parents, carrying instructions to build a baby. As the embryo grows, cells read these instructions to form organs, tissues, and all the parts of the body. Each type of cell reads a specific part of the DNA recipe, like different chapters in a cookbook.

As cells grow and divide, they send and receive messages to communicate with each other, working together to build the baby. These messages, or signals, tell cells which genes to turn on or off. This helps each cell develop its unique role—like how a skin cell is different from a stomach cell, even though they both have the same DNA. Over time, these signals shape the cell's identity and function, guiding a simple stem cell to become any one of hundreds of different cell types in the body.

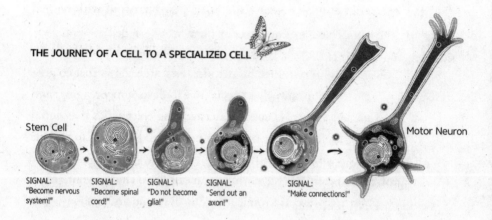

THE JOURNEY OF A CELL TO A SPECIALIZED CELL

Stem Cell

Motor Neuron

SIGNAL:
"Become nervous
system!"

SIGNAL:
"Become spinal
cord!"

SIGNAL:
"Do not become
glia!"

SIGNAL:
"Send out an
axon!"

SIGNAL:
"Make connections!"

As a person grows from childhood to adulthood, a variety of factors start shaping the DNA's epigenetic "memory." These factors include social interactions, environment, physical activity, diet, and more. They send messages to cells, guiding them through important stages of life, like puberty and menopause. Even in old age, cells respond to these signals, helping maintain the body by renewing skin and blood cells and repairing tissues. Throughout your life, these signals continuously influence your cells, turning certain genes on or off as needed. This flexible system allows your body to adapt to changes in your environment, ensuring your cells keep up with your life.[94]

Change Your Cells

You can help your cells adapt to the challenges in their environment and the world at large so that they can thrive in nearly any situation. The cells in Eric's body, in giraffes and trees and their interconnected networks, in flatworms, and in each of you have the miraculous ability to adeptly respond to their unique challenges. Your DNA provides the blueprints for the way your physical cells are built, but the experiences (signals) you provide your cells determines everything else. Diseases such as heart disease, type 2 diabetes, and even chronic diseases like cancer are simply problems with the cells. Following the Cell Well model and recommendations, you can protect your cells from challenges and reboot them when needed, potentially side-stepping disease entirely.

Chapter 3
Keyhole Concepts

- ✦ You don't have to change your DNA to change the way your cells and body behave.
- ✦ Your DNA programs the development of your cells, but the experiences you provide your cells determine everything else.
- ✦ The food you eat, the water you drink, the soil you stand on, the air you breathe, and the energetic world you live in can give you an umbrella of protection from the inevitable challenges your cells will face.
- ✦ Your body and cells are changeable, and that is why you can take charge of your wellness.
- ✦ Thankfully, challenged cells can return to normal function when you work to reboot the epigenome.
- ✦ Disease is not inevitable. You can help your cells adapt to and thrive in nearly any situation.
- ✦ Signals come from inside the cell, from neighboring cells, or from the outside world (environment).
- ✦ If cells are given what they need to be healthy, they can pass that on to the next cells as they divide. Thus, if you can make one cell healthy, you can make every cell healthy.

CHAPTER 4

Wellness Combined

According to a World Health Day 2022 poll of two thousand respondents, many people reported that the thing holding them back from a healthier life was simply that they didn't know the best actions to take to be healthy.[95] They felt overwhelmed by too many options and didn't know how to choose what was right for them.

Have you felt this way, too?

What Should You Do to Keep Your Cells and Body Well?

The internet and social media are filled with conflicting health messages. For example, some sites say eating less fat is best for your heart, but eating more fat and fewer carbs is the way to go to maintain a healthy weight. Some "influencers" say coffee is good for your brain, while others warn it can make you anxious. Similar tangles surround gluten, sun exposure, and even celery. Trendy health ideas like detox diets and superfoods often rely more on hype than science. So, what health camp should you belong to in order to stay well?

You've learned about cells, how the Cell Well model works, and that you can keep your cells well despite inevitable challenges. Now it's time to learn how to sort through health messages and options. Using the four areas of the Cell Well model, you will learn how to evaluate different health options and understand what they will provide for your cells. You'll find you don't have to choose between traditional knowledge or modern Western medicine, the "camps" medicine has been divided into today. There is value in both types of medicine, and together they are better than each one alone.

A Fork in the Road

When I got sick, I found myself at a very difficult fork in the road. My grandfather was a doctor, my father was a dentist, and I had followed in their footsteps, learning and practicing in the modern Western medicine framework. Unfortunately, this medical model didn't provide me with the tools that I needed to stay well and prevent illness in the first place, nor was it giving me the answers that I needed to get well once I was sick. When I found out that my health problems stemmed from mercury poisoning, I started to question modern Western medicine and my education in general. If I hadn't been taught about the dangers of mercury, what else was missing from my education? Frustrated and feeling like I only knew half of the story, I ventured onto a new path, looking further back than the last 150 years of "modern medicine." What I found surprised me in many ways.

Historically, traditional health-care practitioners provided wellness and disease care using natural substances like plants, animals, and minerals. As I learned about these traditional practices and started using them personally on my path back to wellness, some of these new beliefs filtered into my dental practice. I started talking to patients about mercury and what I was doing to heal my cells, and shared why I was removing mercury in a new, safer way. The changes I was making soon gained me the reputation in professional circles as the "crazy" dentist. I didn't know the kind of controversy I was stirring up until, at lunch at a prestigious dental conference, the conversation turned to questionable practices in dentistry. One of the dentists at my table laughed and shared that a practitioner in his office building wore a hazmat suit to remove "silver" fillings. What he didn't know is that I had begun using similar protection when removing mercury-containing "silver" fillings.

Everyone else at the table scoffed and shook their heads, and I swallowed hard and spoke up. I asked if I could share my story. After I told them about my experiences with these fillings, those very educated colleagues were embarrassed and apologized. I told them no apology was necessary, and that I had shared simply because I wanted to spare them and others in the profession from the same health challenges I struggled with. The protective approaches I had adopted are frequently viewed as outdated, primitive, or "pre-scientific," no longer needed by practitioners of modern, scientifically grounded medicine.[96] Many of my traditional medicine practitioner friends have also faced similar professional prejudices.

But interestingly, public opinion seems to be going the opposite direction. The demand for traditional medicine remains strong globally, and my dental practice and many others are bursting at the seams with patients desperate to get well and thrilled to find practitioners who are willing to try all kinds of approaches to help them, and their cells, stay well.

You Don't Have to Choose

Traditional medicine (also known as alternative or folk medicine) encompasses a variety of wellness practices that have been used around the world for millennia. Because of the diversity in practices and methodologies, some have found traditional medicine challenging to classify, but the World Health Organization has recently defined it as "the sum total of the knowledge, skills, and practices based on the theories, beliefs, and experiences indigenous to different cultures, whether explainable or not."

Though modern Western medicine has incorporated some of these traditional practices, its approaches are scientifically based and supported by statistical research.[97] Both types of medicine can gain from the other, and medicine is better when they are used in tandem. Medicine, after all, is the sum of all the knowledge and skills and experiences of everyone working together throughout history to help us be well collectively and individually.

Throughout history, people took charge of their wellness by applying inherited wisdom and wellness practices passed down through generations. Families relied on medicinal plants, traditional wellness practices like meditation and acupuncture, and collective communal knowledge. The village healer was one of the most respected figures in the community, keeping those they cared for well with nature's gifts. But as time passed, health care shifted to a new type of practitioner in a new type of medicine we call "modern." The nineteenth and twentieth centuries witnessed the rise of antibiotics, vaccines, and surgical innovations, which transformed the healing landscape. The allure of urban life drew people away from their regional roots and family homes, which led to a widespread shift in where people turned for answers to health concerns. Traditional agrarian societies merged into an urban bustle, bringing a new set of challenges. Diets changed, stress levels rose, and exposure to environmental pollutants like smoke and factory chemicals increased, leading to a surge in health issues like asthma. These ailments seemed to require more help than traditional remedies could provide. While traditional medicine had played a crucial role in whole-body wellness and prevention, the acute and chronic conditions stemming from modern industrial life were new challenges. People turned to pharmaceuticals, surgical procedures, and other medical technologies that were developed in response to new diseases and triggers.

In these new urban societies, doctors began to specialize, giving rise to a different doctor for every part of the body. Technological marvels further fueled the transformation of the medical system. New medical instruments and pharmaceuticals like penicillin offered precision in diagnosis and treatment of diseases. Cultural attitudes shifted, and the narrative around health evolved. Seeking out professional medical advice, versus seeking out knowledge passed down from elders, became the norm. Health insurance, a new concept introduced during the Great Depression, flourished post–World War II. Intended to attract and retain workers, these "benefits" provided a financial safety net for some, allowing them to turn to medical institutions instead of relying on traditional knowledge and home remedies for a broad range of health concerns.[98] Today there is also the added blessing and curse of the internet. While it has empowered individuals to learn more about how their bodies work, it has also ushered in an era of "cyberchondria," where information overload from Dr. Google has led to an even greater reliance on medical professionals.

While we benefit from advancements in medical science, it is important to remain engaged in and responsible for our health. The good news is that you don't have to choose one kind of medicine or the other. The debate between them can largely be boiled down to a lack of understanding about the value both methodologies contribute. A balance of modern medical innovations combined with traditional wisdom forms the foundation of the Cell Well model of care.

The goal of all health care is the same: to help people stay well. Modern and traditional medicine are stronger and better together.

The Coming Together of Medicine

My first tentative steps toward practicing this combined wellness approach happened long before social media, Google searches, or AI tools existed. At that time, information lived in books and libraries, magazines, and at the kitchen tables of friends and family. Figuring out how to stop getting a stomachache after every meal was first on my list of ailments to find solutions for.

As you learned in chapter 1, according to the Cell Well model, gut cells need to be supplied with all the nutrients they require to work correctly. Since I had no idea how to supply my gut cells with the nutrients they needed, at the suggestion of friends, I decided to do an experiment: I emptied my cupboards of everything packaged, processed, white in color, and full of the Standard American Diet trifecta: sugar, fat, and salt. It was shocking to find how few foods this left for my young family to eat. I refilled our pantry with foods labeled "organic," hoping that the label made whatever was in the box better for us somehow. My husband and I chuckle as we remember the case of "organic" gummy bears we bought for our kids. We were struggling to make sense of labels and marketing promises on food and simply trying to do the best for our family. As we continued to learn about cells and fuel and what really made a difference for our energy and wellness levels, we realized those package labels don't carry as much weight as we once thought. After all, humankind has been eating "organic" for centuries! The label alone didn't ensure wellness; the energy in the food was what my gut cells and body needed. Instead of, "Is it organic?" my new question became, "What does this food supply for my cells?"

Plant Medicine for Gut Health

Chew soothing licorice tablets to relieve the pain of a stomach ache.

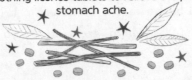

Add tumeric to favorite dishes to decrease gut inflammation.

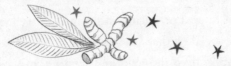

Drink chamomile tea at night to calm the body and gut.

Use peppermint essential oil beadlets for immediate relief when away from home.

The next things my gut cells needed were *support* and *security*. Becoming less enchanted with finding the right package or label led me to foods and medicine that didn't come in a package or have labels at all: herbal or plant medicines. Also called botanical or phytomedicine, this kind of medicine is made using plants' seeds, berries, roots, leaves, bark, and/or flowers to improve wellness, and is practiced in every country around the globe. I started incorporating plants into my day and meals. I tried the steps listed on page 80.

Once I realized that the plants already in my garden and spice cabinet could give my gut cells the support and security they needed, I started intentionally adding them as "medicine" to the meals I cooked.

✦ Garlic added to mashed potatoes helped to protect my cells and kill off any parasites or other microbes that were impacting my gut health.

✦ My afternoon snack of apples and dates gave my gut fiber and pre-biotics, which support the growth and activity of good bacteria in the digestive system. Those good bacteria made it easier for me to digest food. The fiber also fed good bacteria and helped food move through my digestive system faster, helping with the discomfort, bloating, and constipation I had been struggling with.

I was feeding my cells what they needed straight from the kitchen and garden. As I widened my exploration to the brambles and bushes in the hills around my home, I was shocked to find plants all around me that could support and secure all my cells, helping me feel well and avoid getting sick!

Let's learn about the origins of some of these "modern" medicines that aren't actually that modern at all.

Medicine Comes from Nature

Did you know aspirin comes from tree bark? Let's follow its development from tree to bottle:

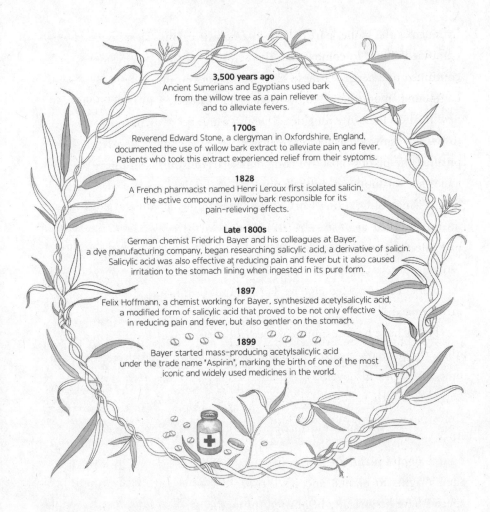

3,500 years ago
Ancient Sumerians and Egyptians used bark
from the willow tree as a pain reliever
and to alleviate fevers.

1700s
Reverend Edward Stone, a clergyman in Oxfordshire, England,
documented the use of willow bark extract to alleviate pain and fever.
Patients who took this extract experienced relief from their syptoms.

1828
A French pharmacist named Henri Leroux first isolated salicin,
the active compound in willow bark responsible for its
pain-relieving effects.

Late 1800s
German chemist Friedrich Bayer and his colleagues at Bayer,
a dye manufacturing company, began researching salicylic acid, a derivative of salicin.
Salicylic acid was also effective at reducing pain and fever but it also caused
irritation to the stomach lining when ingested in its pure form.

1897
Felix Hoffmann, a chemist working for Bayer, synthesized acetylsalicylic acid,
a modified form of salicylic acid that proved to be not only effective
in reducing pain and fever, but also gentler on the stomach.

1899
Bayer started mass-producing acetylsalicylic acid
under the trade name "Aspirin", marking the birth of one of the most
iconic and widely used medicines in the world.

The A in "aspirin" is for acetyl, and "spirin" comes from *Spiraea*, the genus of plants from which salicin was originally extracted. Aspirin quickly gained popularity and widespread use due to its efficacy and relatively low cost. Its pain-relieving, anti-inflammatory, and fever-reducing properties revolutionized the treatment of various conditions, including headaches, arthritis, and heart diseases. Aspirin has become a staple in medicine cabinets worldwide and is an example of the success that comes when modern and traditional medicine converge.

Today's preferred treatment for malaria is a perfect example of this combination. In the 1960s, malaria was wreaking havoc and claiming lives across the globe, particularly in tropical regions. Despite worldwide combined efforts to combat the disease, new, medication-resistant strains continued to emerge. Chinese scientist Tu Youyou tested compound after compound, more than 240,000 total, before turning to traditional Chinese medical literature for clues. There, she and her team found a reference to sweet wormwood as a fever treatment. They meticulously extracted and purified the plant's bioactive component, artemisinin, and found a medicine that was nothing short of miraculous. Unlike previous antimalarial drugs, which often didn't work against certain strains of the disease, artemisinin worked against every strain and swiftly killed the parasite that had infected people. Today, artemisinin is endorsed by the World Health Organization as a frontline treatment for the disease, and Tu was awarded the Nobel Prize in Medicine for her groundbreaking contributions to the medical field.[99]

Plants have been a source of medical treatments for millennia. Quinine, the primary treatment for malaria for more than three centuries preceding Tu's discovery, originated from the bark of cinchona trees, native to South America. The use of a plant called foxglove in ancient times paved the way for development of the modern heart medication digoxin, and morphine and codeine were initially derived from the opium poppy plant. In fact, a quarter of today's pharmaceuticals trace their origins to plants, and it's estimated that seventy thousand plant species have historically been used for medicinal purposes.[100] Before the arrival of modern times, these traditional medicines were the foundation of health-care systems worldwide. Even if healers didn't understand cells or energy or know why their methods worked, what mattered was that they did work.

Tu, Hoffmann, Bayer, and many other scientists have combined scientific methods with knowledge of nature to improve modern medicine, and in fact, much of the modern medicine you use today comes from traditional medicines your great-grandmothers used. The pills, like aspirin, that fill your medicine cabinet are largely derived from plants, fungi, minerals, or other elements from the natural world.

The Meeting of Medicines

These are interesting examples of how traditional and modern medicine can converge. Can this happen more often? Can they come together more effectively? Let's turn to nature again for an example.

Years ago, I visited a fascinating natural phenomenon called the Meeting of Waters in Brazil, where two distinct rivers, the Rio Negro and the Rio Solimões, converge to form the Amazon River. What makes these rivers' convergence unique is that the two rivers have different colors, temperatures, and speeds of flow. The Rio Negro has dark, almost black, water due to the tannins from decomposing plants in the surrounding forests, while the Rio Solimões has lighter-colored, muddy water due to soil and other sediment picked up along its journey. I took a boat out to this meeting place, and it looked like Coke meeting chocolate milk. When the two rivers come together, they flow side by side for several kilometers without mixing, which creates a striking visual contrast. Eventually, the differences in temperature, speed, and density in the rivers help the two rivers gradually mix as their currents and turbulence interact. Together, they create the massive, powerful Amazon River. Just like the two rivers flowing together to create the Amazon, it's time for a "meeting of medicines." Traditional and modern medicine have been traveling side by side for some time, and now it's time for them to come together to create a stronger, more powerful medical system that keeps cells well and prevents disease from occurring.

When I was struggling to find answers for my own health challenges, this idea of combining the best in all methods and approaches felt very right to me. I began to study the roots of many different medicines and approaches. Research led me to ancient practices like Native American traditional medicine, German herbalism, traditional Chinese medicine, and Ayurveda from India. Similarities between all of them helped me realize that much knowledge was shared across continents and cultures. In ancient times, Greek philosophers like Pythagoras and Democritus ventured to India in pursuit of knowledge. Hippocrates, a student of Democritus, proposed a model for understanding the human body which looked very similar to the Indian Ayurvedic model. He shared his new model with Roman contemporaries. Medicines, herbs, and spices traveled along the Silk Road to China and along Roman trade routes, eventually finding their way to Spain, Italy, the Netherlands, and other European countries.[101] Today, many of these practices have been validated by modern science. Here are some you might recognize:

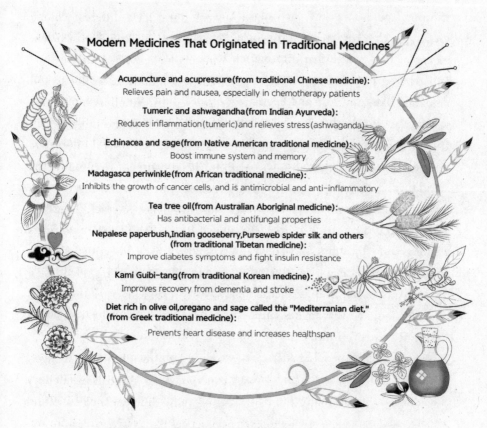

Modern Medicines That Originated in Traditional Medicines

Acupuncture and acupressure (from traditional Chinese medicine):
Relieves pain and nausea, especially in chemotherapy patients

Tumeric and ashwagandha (from Indian Ayurveda):
Reduces inflammation (tumeric) and relieves stress (ashwaganda)

Echinacea and sage (from Native American traditional medicine):
Boost immune system and memory

Madagasca periwinkle (from African traditional medicine):
Inhibits the growth of cancer cells, and is antimicrobial and anti-inflammatory

Tea tree oil (from Australian Aboriginal medicine):
Has antibacterial and antifungal properties

Nepalese paperbush, Indian gooseberry, Purseweb spider silk and others (from traditional Tibetan medicine):
Improve diabetes symptoms and fight insulin resistance

Kami Guibi-tang (from traditional Korean medicine):
Improves recovery from dementia and stroke

Diet rich in olive oil, oregano and sage called the "Mediterranian diet," (from Greek traditional medicine):
Prevents heart disease and increases healthspan

Sources for illustration: 102, 103, 104, 105, 106, 107, 108, 109, 110

As stated earlier, there is no reason to limit yourself to Western medicine or to one traditional medicine approach. Combining them gives your cells, and you, the "best of all worlds."

The Cell Well Model Is a Global
Model of Medicine

As much as I loved studying wellness traditions from around the world, I was disappointed to find that, even after extensive research, I was no closer to an approach that was easy to understand and easy to apply. It was all too complex and complicated.

For example, as I studied Ayurveda from India, I learned that my "constitution," or the way my particular mind and body work, is called Vata-Pitta type. Unfortunately, most people, me included, don't know what that means or how to use that information to be well. In Western herbalism, I discovered I needed to choose herbal remedies that were "alterative" or detoxing, like dandelion and licorice root. But I didn't know how much to use, if I should take them in a capsule or tea, and what effect I should expect from using them. My Western medical diagnoses were irritable bowel syndrome, thoracic outlet syndrome, and heavy metal toxicity. I could understand these diagnoses, but on their own, they left me no closer to a solution.

Fascinated, as well as overwhelmed and still not well, I decided that what I needed to do was create a simple, integrated approach and method of care that everyone (including me) could understand and use. As I sorted all the information into categories, a pattern started to emerge, shown on page 87.

As you can see, all these methodologies use the elements of the earth for classification, and that makes sense. The earth and her elements have been a part of existence through every century and era of human life. They are a constant that all people understand; we all live on the earth, eat what she produces, drink her water, and breathe her air. These elements cycle annually through seasons, allowing planting, growing, harvesting, and rejuvenating to all happen in turn.

Humans have long recognized the value of these elements and cyclical seasons in health and wellness, as shown by the element-based classifications from civilizations across the globe. There are few things that all humans, living on any continent, in any culture, and speaking any language, share and understand more than the earth, the elements, and the seasons. This is why they are at the core of the Cell Well model. This universal system of classification weaves traditional and modern medicine together into a simple, intuitive lifelong approach to wellness.

Traditional Medicine Classification Systems

Ayurvedic medicine categorizes individuals into three constitutional types (doshas):
1. Vata (Air and Ether)
2. Pitta (Fire and Water)
3. Kapha (Earth and Water)

In traditional Chinese medicine there are five elements:
1. Wood
2. Fire
3. Earth
4. Metal
5. Water

Tibetan medicine, or Sowa Rigpa, incorporates the concept of three humours:
1. Loong (Air)
2. MKhris-pa (Fire)
3. Bad-kan (Earth and Water)

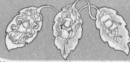

Japanese medical systems, including Kampo, categorize medicinal herbs according to their energetic properties:
1. Heating (Fire)
2. Cooling (Air)
3. Drying (Earth)
4. Moistening (Water)

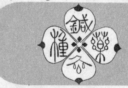

Western and European herbalism and folk medicine classifies plants according to elemental properties:
1. Hot (Fire)
2. Cold (Air)
3. Moist (Water)
4. Dry (Earth)

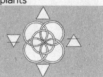

Elements and Seasons Combined Classification System

In the Cell Well model, each of the five elements of the earth correlates with a season of the earth: Spring/Plants, Summer/Fire, Harvest/Earth, Fall/Air, and Winter/Water. These will each be explored in depth in Part Two of the book. In Part Three, you will then learn how to use this model to create personalized wellness formulas. These classifications and formulas are an owner's manual for your cells and body, giving you all the information you need to be well.

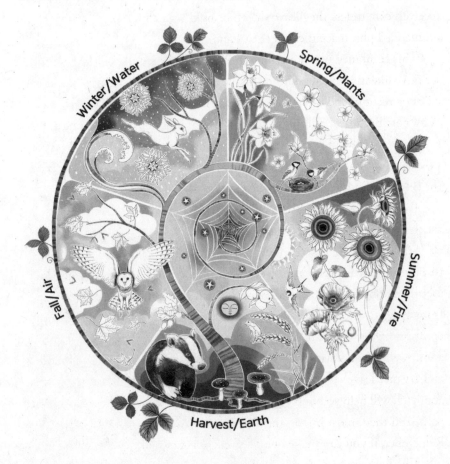

Cell Well Formulas

Be prepared to tweak your thinking about what health care and wellness care look like. When starting down the path of combined traditional and modern medicine, you might feel a tendency to veer to the modern side and start looking for prescriptions for herbs and other natural substances as if they were pharmaceutical drugs. You might be tempted to Google "what herb/pharmaceutical/remedy do I use for this symptom/diagnosis/condition."

You need to break this pattern. Doctors prescribe pharmaceuticals because it is the "standard of care" today, but also because it's the treatment and solution patients have come to expect. Many people don't feel they have received care unless they leave the office holding a slip of paper with a recommended pharmaceutical in their hand.

This combined path and the Cell Well model supporting it are not prescriptive like modern Western medicine, and you will not find specific remedies or recommendations for each ailment or health challenge you have. Why not? Because a pill might address a symptom you have right now, but it doesn't usually address what is happening to your cells that led to you experiencing that symptom. This model empowers you to stay well, from the cells outward, regardless of the diagnosis or symptom.

Does this make sense? Does it make you nervous that it will be too much work or won't be effective?

Stay with me. After talking with thousands of people, and living through my own experience, I know the feeling of overwhelm when you are in the middle of a health crisis. You have information coming at you from every direction, and you aren't sure what to do. Compounding the confusion, your body and mind simply aren't working their best when you are unwell. I know what this feels like. Don't worry. The Cell Well model and I won't leave you without a clear path forward. To the contrary, this approach will help you find the right path, know how to progress down that path, and then, most importantly, never have to return to that path again. Remember, if you can make one cell well, you can make every cell well.

This harkens back to the well-known proverb about fishing: "Give a man a fish, and you feed him for a day. Teach a man to fish, and you feed him for a lifetime." If I recommend a pill or remedy for you, it will help you be well for today. That's not good enough. The Cell Well model will teach you wellness for a lifetime.

The Cell Well model will teach you fundamentals and formulas for wellness rather than recipes to cure diseases.

Still worried or doubting? Let me explain it another way. I love to cook, and for years, I would follow recipes to the letter, worrying that if I strayed from the recommended ingredients and instructions, the meal would be a flop. Many people have been trained to treat their health care similarly. You want the perfect recipe for your health right now. The perfect supplement or superfood or exercise regimen. The problem is that if a new health concern or challenge comes along, you will be starting at square one again. That's reactive, not proactive, and doesn't bring wellness at all. I have since been taught the fundamentals and formulas for cooking, how to make food taste good, how to season correctly, how and when to use different cooking methods, and more. I still love recipes, but now that I really know how to cook, I use them for ideas rather than instruction. This model teaches you how to "cook" and address wellness at any age and stage and situation.

My family learned this in an interesting way. As I was going through my wellness journey, my husband Steve had some unexpected benefits as well. He had struggled for years with painful and frequent canker sores in his mouth, headaches, and a chronic congested nose. As a dentist, the cankers were in my area of expertise, but I had been taught that canker sores are "idiopathic" or without known cause. As we searched for possible triggers, we noticed that after he ate Reese's peanut butter cups (something he loved), the cankers seemed to get worse. For nearly ten years, Steve avoided his beloved Reese's candy, peanut butter, and all other nuts. It seemed to help some, but the cankers didn't completely go away. Throughout those same ten years, he wasn't what most would call sick, but he fell into a pattern of covering up symptoms. He carried a small container with ibuprofen and nasal decongestant in his pants pocket, always ready to tamp down a headache or clear a stuffy nose. This became his habit until his diet changed along with mine.

- ✦ For breakfast, we swapped out the processed and sweetened cereal and milk, pancakes, and maple-flavored corn syrup (very common American breakfast foods), for a blended green smoothie made of spinach, fruit, and water.
- ✦ We substituted our go-to pre-packaged and frozen lunch foods like burritos and pasta for whole, unprocessed staple foods, including vegetables and rice.

✦ We cut out soda and candy, so Steve started making a drink with chia seeds, lime juice, and honey in water to drink when he wanted a "treat."

These food changes, along with using herbal remedies where he had previously relied on pharmaceuticals, resulted in Steve having few to no canker sores, even while eating nuts, and losing fifteen pounds. His headaches and stuffy nose mysteriously disappeared.

Which one thing on this list of changes cured his canker sores? Were the green smoothies for breakfast the answer? Was it the rice and veggies for lunch? Maybe it was the herbal anti-inflammatory that he now had at hand but didn't have to use often. Steve's story illustrates the challenge of the "recipe for wellness" model. There wasn't just one thing that did the trick. We believe his improved health was a result of a combination of the changes we were making. More important than receiving a prescription to mask symptoms was creating a formula that would provide what his cells needed to get well and stay well.

Looking back, we see we were checking off all the Cell Well boxes without realizing it! Here's how our changes fit into this model:

 Supply: Steve's old go-to breakfast started his cells off with very few usable nutrients for the day. Inflamed from the sugar, his head ached, and his sinuses were stuffy. In contrast, the green smoothies were full to the brim with nutrients that lowered his inflammation.

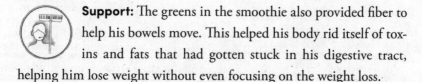 **Support:** The greens in the smoothie also provided fiber to help his bowels move. This helped his body rid itself of toxins and fats that had gotten stuck in his digestive tract, helping him lose weight without even focusing on the weight loss.

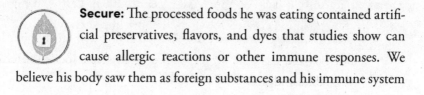 **Secure:** The processed foods he was eating contained artificial preservatives, flavors, and dyes that studies show can cause allergic reactions or other immune responses. We believe his body saw them as foreign substances and his immune system

began to fight them. As the fighting continued nonstop for years, his immune system became weary and confused and started injuring his own body, especially his mouth. Some researchers believe that canker sores occur because of this misguided immune system response, and because of our experience, I agree. Once he stopped giving his immune system so many things to fight, Steve's canker sores went away.

Signal: The frozen, processed meals he ate for lunch were devoid of electrons, leaving his signaling systems without the energy they needed to communicate well. With an increase of electrons from the vegetables in his new lunches, his systems all picked up the pace, leading to less inflammation, weight loss, and a general feeling of wellness.

Using the Elements and Seasons of Wellness

This all probably sounds good in theory, but you might be asking how it applies to you. Let's take a very simple example that most everyone has experienced at some time in their life: the common cold.

It's now time to learn more about the Elements that will provide all your cells' needs. This will be the focus of Part Two. In Part Three, you'll learn about the Seasons that guide how and when you use the Elements. There isn't a starting or stopping place in the Seasonal cycle or a right or wrong place to begin. The Seasons and their Elements flow from one to another, and you will find yourself moving through them fluidly as you identify what your cells need.

To find the Season you should start on, you can pause here to take the Seasons of Wellness Assessment found in chapter 11—or you can dive straight into the Elements of Wellness in Part Two and take the Assessment when you get to that chapter. (The Assessment, both in PDF and digital form, can also be found at www.resources.livingwellbook.com.)

Example: Treating the Common Cold

Modern Methods   **Wellness Methods**

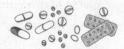

Take pills to treat symptoms.

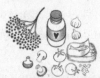

Elderberry, nutrient-rich foods, and vitamins to strengthen immune health.

Give your body time to heal.

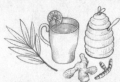

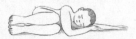

Rest until symptoms are gone.

Eat medicinal herbs and food (like eucalyptus, tumeric, honey, or lemon ginger tea) to relieve symptoms.

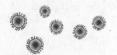

Wait for next time you "catch" a cold.

The body is stronger and better prepared to resist a cold next time!

Chapter 4
Keyhole Concepts

✦ As a society, we have gradually transitioned from being able to care for our health and wellness independently to a shaky dependence on professionals and the modern medical system.

✦ Much of modern medicine comes from traditional medicine practices and practitioners. The pills and potions, like aspirin, that fill our medicine cabinets, are largely derived from plants, herbs, minerals, or other elements in our natural world.

✦ Medicine is the sum of all the knowledge and skills and experiences of everyone working to help you and me be well.

+ The goal of all health care is the same: to help people stay well. In working toward this goal, modern and traditional medicine are stronger and better together.

+ The Cell Well model combines traditional and modern Western medicine approaches and transforms them into usable, timely, personal guides for better energy and health today and for the duration of your life.

+ Staying well is as simple as providing the correct building blocks for your cells to operate, heal, and regenerate efficiently and effectively, and those building blocks are found in the Elements and Seasons of the earth.

PART TWO

....

Elements of Wellness

In Part One of *Living Well with Dr. Michelle*, you learned that wellness is about your cells having what they need to stay well so you can live the life you want. Throughout this section, you will learn where all the Elements that your cells need to stay well come from and how to tap into the limitless supply of the Elements that the earth provides. Each chapter in this section will highlight one of the Elements—fire, plants, earth, air, and water.

We'll delve into the rich history and scientific foundations of the featured Element. We will examine how ancient healers harnessed its properties and how modern medicine has adapted these practices to enhance therapeutic outcomes. You will learn about the Elements' physiological impact on the cells and body and discover practical ways to incorporate them into your daily life to optimize cellular energy and promote wellness. The goal: to equip you with an understanding of each Element's potential to boost your energy levels and support your overall wellness.

CHAPTER 5

Fire

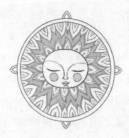

Do you feel like you are perpetually running on empty? If so, you're in good company. A staggering three out of five adults in the U.S. report feeling more drained today than ever before.[111]

This problem resonates among stretched students, multitasking parents, overextended professionals, and weary grandparents alike. It seems the quest for more energy is a universal one, with an astounding 85 percent of Americans reaching for caffeine daily to stoke their energy.[112] But what if the solution to having more energy can't be found in another cup of coffee or a fleeting afternoon nap?

The real answer lies deep within your cells. Every cell in your body is a powerhouse of energy, diligently working to keep you moving, thinking, and thriving. This cellular energy is responsible for everything from moving your muscles to digesting your lunch, and it perpetually keeps your brain buzzing and your heart pumping. Essentially, cellular energy is the unsung hero behind every thought you think and every step you take. Yet this energy isn't just floating around for you to "find"; it's generated from the Five Elements of the earth. The food you eat, the air you breathe, the water you drink—all of these are transformed into cellular energy that fuels your body, no caffeine required. Understanding the relationship between your cellular energy and your overall energy is a game-changer.

Cellular energy is known as the "fire" Element in traditional medicine. You will learn how to support your cells in transforming natural fuel into batteries full of energy called adenosine triphosphate (ATP) and how cell signals work to help you stay well. Next time you feel a mid-afternoon slump coming on, remember the secret to boundless energy doesn't come from a can or a cup, but from caring for the natural energy factories inside each of your cells. Fuel them well, and they will power you through your day and your life. In this chapter, you will learn about the options you have for cellular fuel: carbohydrates, fats, and proteins, and how your cells use each of them in the Cell Well model. Through integrated systems and signals, your cells keep your body energized. Let's dive into how it all works.

Cellular Power Generation

There is a lot of debate online about the best fuel or food for your body (much of which will be cleared up in subsequent chapters), but little talk or knowledge about *how* that fuel is used to make your cells' energy. The Cell Well model, with its four divisions, described below, will help you understand how your cells generate and use energy:

+ **Supply:** Plants, the earth, air, and water all have energy-containing molecules in them that supply your cells and body with fuel. Higher quality fuel leads to better (and more) energy created.

+ **Support and Secure:** Cells take the different types of fuel in, sort them, process them, and convert them into a usable power source. When your cells' internal processes are clear of toxins or pollutants, they work efficiently, and you get as much energy as you need out of your cellular power generators.

+ **Signal:** Your cells receive external signals from the surrounding environment and internal signals about needs from the cell itself, and using these signals, create the needed energy. When these cellular signals are received, your internal power generators work hard and keep your cells pumping out more energy when needed.

When your cells have the right fuel, they produce energy. When they produce energy, you have energy—it's very simple. The great news is that you can learn to keep your cellular power plants working at full efficiency, so you feel great and have the energy you need to live well.

Supply: The Fuel for Your Cells

Life runs on chemical energy. Where do your cells get this chemical energy? The answer lies in the dynamic duo of food and oxygen. Here's how it works: every time you take a bite of food, you're not just satisfying your hunger, you're fueling the powerhouse within your cells known as mitochondria. These tiny structures are where the magic happens. They transform nutrients into the chemical energy that powers every cell in your body. Similarly, each breath you take isn't just about filling your lungs; it's about feeding oxygen to your mitochondria to boost this energy transformation process. It's like throwing gasoline on a flame, significantly ramping up your energy production.[113]

This combination of nutrients and oxygen that fuels your body is a perfect example of biophysics in action. While nutrition science often zooms in on the biochemical makeup of what you consume—the vitamins, minerals, proteins, carbohydrates, and fats—biophysics shifts the focus to what your cells can do with those molecules. It explores the potential energy you can extract from your food. Consider this: if you plant an apple seed, it can grow into a tree that not only lives but thrives, producing bushels of apples for many seasons. Plant a kernel of corn, and it shoots up into a stalk, yielding ears packed with hundreds more kernels. But what happens if you plant a processed apple snack bar or a corn chip? Nothing. These processed foods, stripped of their natural vitality and no longer capable of growth, illustrate a lost potential to generate and sustain energy.

How Our Cells Use Food To Generate Power

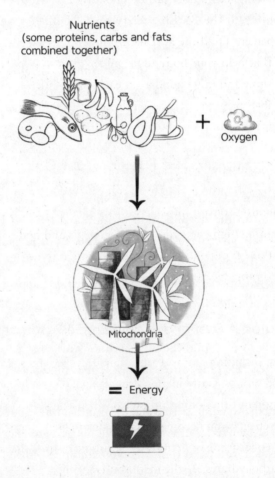

Nutrients
(some proteins, carbs and fats
combined together)

+ Oxygen

Mitochondria

= Energy

This is where an understanding of biophysics comes into play. It can guide you in choosing the types of fuel that will maximize your energy levels. In the upcoming chapters on the Elements and Seasons of Wellness, you'll find out how you can apply these principles of biophysics to super-charge every cell in your body, enhancing your energy and vitality. Every function in your body and cells requires the energy generated within the microscopic mitochondrial "powerhouses" inside your cells.

Organs or tissues with particularly high energy needs, like the heart and liver, have a higher number of mitochondria per cell than other types of cells. According to the British Society for Cell Biology, mitochondria fill nearly 40 percent of all the area within heart muscle cells.[114] Similarly, the liver cells that help your body filter out toxins and waste can have up to one to two thousand mitochondria in each cell. Without mitochondria, you couldn't move, breathe, eat, or even think; your mitochondria make life possible. But to function properly, mitochondria need to be provided with the correct fuel. You can have a perfectly constructed power plant, but if you have poor-quality fuel with little "energy potential" in it, the output of the plant will be suboptimal. The food you eat supplies the fuel that your body's mitochondria convert into energy, so a balanced diet is very import-ant for maintaining high energy levels in your cells and body.

There are three types of fuel that your mitochondria can use: carbohy-drates, fats, and proteins.

Carbohydrates: A Fast and Highly Efficient Source of Fuel

Carbohydrates, including grains, fruits, dairy, and legumes, are one of the most basic food groups. Carbohydrate (sugar) metabolism keeps your brain and nervous system functioning properly. When your blood sugar is low, you notice the effects: you become irritable, disoriented, and lethargic, and find it hard to concentrate or perform even simple tasks. Glucose and other sugars from carbohydrates are the main source of energy for many types of cells, particularly the brain.

Some Facts About Carbohydrates as Fuel

✦ Less oxygen is required to burn carbohydrates than fats, making carbohydrates very important during high-intensity exercise when the body cannot process enough oxygen to meet its needs.

✦ To burn fats effectively, your body must break down a certain amount of carbohydrates. If you consume too few carbohydrates, it limits fat metabolism.

✦ Eating enough carbohydrates allows the body to use proteins to build, maintain, and repair body tissues including muscle, hormones, enzymes, and neurotransmitters.

✦ Glucose can be stored as glycogen in the liver and muscles and can be rapidly metabolized to produce ATP for short-term needs.

Fats: An Energy-Dense Fuel

Fats provide a concentrated source of energy, with each gram of fat providing more than twice the potential energy (calories) as proteins or carbohydrates.

Some Facts About Fats as Fuel

✦ Fats help fuel your body through long-duration activities and times when energy needs to be sustained over an extended period.

✦ During fasting or over a longer time with limited food, the body relies on stored fat for energy. Over time, this can lead to loss of your body's fat stores.

Protein: The Last Option for Fuel

Proteins are primarily used for structure and for specific functions in your body such as building muscle. They are present in tissues like muscles, organs, and blood, where they serve essential roles in growth, repair, and regulation. Proteins aren't often used for fuel. When they are, it leads to loss of lean body mass and impairs vital functions.

Some Facts About Protein as Fuel

✦ When carbohydrate and fat stores are gone, your body will break down skeletal muscle protein. The glucose created when this happens can supply up to 15 percent of the energy your body needs.

✦ Protein metabolism for energy is the least efficient of the three types. Amino acids in proteins must undergo complex processes to be converted into ATP, making the energy yield relatively low compared to fats and carbohydrates.

Support and Secure: Metabolic Pathways

Carbohydrates, fats, and proteins all store energy in a concentrated, stable form and are used by the cells to make energy in different ways. At the end of finely tuned metabolic processes, they all ultimately become molecules of chemical energy called ATP. An ATP molecule is like a rechargeable battery: when broken apart, its energy can be used by the cell, and then the "worn-out battery" can be recharged by reattaching new molecules. How many of these batteries do your cells and body use? A single cell uses about ten million ATP molecules per second and recycles all its ATP molecules about every twenty to thirty seconds![115] Anytime you need energy to digest your food, to talk, to brush your hair, or to walk around the block, your body uses ATP. In fact, ATP is the only molecule able to provide energy to muscles. ATP itself isn't like a light bulb, radiating energy that can be seen. Instead, it "carries" energy in one of the chemical bonds that holds the molecule together. When this bond is broken, the energy it gives off powers up other cellular processes. This is similar to the glow-in-the-dark chemical light sticks you get at parties or nighttime events. The light stick contains the potential to glow, but the light (energy) isn't released until the stick is bent and broken.

For this ATP to be created, the fuel you eat and breathe must first get to the cells. The first steps in this journey are digestion and absorption. In humans, digestion starts in the mouth and continues in the stomach and small intestine, where carbohydrates, fats, and proteins are broken down into absorbable molecules of glucose, amino acids, and fatty acids. These molecules are absorbed through the lining of the small intestine and end up in the bloodstream. The bloodstream circulates this fuel to cells throughout the body, where it then makes its way through the cell membrane through specialized gates called transport proteins. Once inside the cell, the molecules go through numerous, complex metabolic pathways that eventually lead to the creation of ATP in the cells. All these pathways start with one molecule of fuel and produce anywhere from two to thirty-two molecules of ATP. The number of molecules of ATP that are produced depends on the fuel the cell uses, the kind of cell making the energy, and whether there is oxygen present.

Using Carbohydrates for Fuel

✦ **Step 1—Glycolysis:** This process is like a mini assembly line where glucose, your main energy source from food, gets broken down into smaller molecules through a series of chemical steps. The breakdown of glucose not only releases energy (two ATP) but also provides the starting material for further energy-making processes down the line.

✦ **Step 2—Krebs Cycle:** The broken-down molecules from Step 1 undergo a series of chemical reactions, with molecules swapping partners and rearranging themselves. This cycle creates more energy (two ATP) and molecules that carry electrons to make even more energy in Step 3.

+ **Step 3—Electron Transport Chain:** The electron carrier molecules produced in Step 2 release high-energy electrons, which then move along a chain of special molecules, like a baton being passed in a relay race. As the electrons move along this chain, they create a buildup of potential energy in the mitochondria, which, when combined with oxygen, leads to a surge of energy production, producing up to thirty ATP from one molecule of glucose.

Using Fats for Fuel

+ **Step 1—Beta-oxidation:** Fat molecules are made up of chains of fatty acids that can be broken apart into smaller pieces. These smaller by-products can then be used in the Krebs cycle and electron transport chain, like the carbohydrates described above.
+ **Step 2—Krebs Cycle** (see above)
+ **Step 3—Electron Transport Chain** (see above)

Using Proteins for Fuel

+ **Oxidation of Amino Acids:** When the body needs energy and isn't getting enough from its primary sources, carbohydrates and fats, it breaks down proteins into amino acids for fuel. This typically happens during times of prolonged fasting, intense exercise, or starvation. In these situations, the body starts breaking down its own protein stores, such as muscle tissue, to obtain amino acids for energy production. These amino acids are broken down further to produce ATP. This source of energy is used only if all others aren't available.

Backup Energy Plans

+ **When Oxygen Is Low:**
  • **Lactic Acid Fermentation:** If you are sprinting or working so hard oxygen doesn't have time to get to your muscles, your cells

break glucose in the muscles apart for fast fuel, then convert the by-products into lactic acid, which makes your muscles burn. It's a quick-and-dirty way to make energy without oxygen.

✦ **When Carbohydrates Are Low:**

- **Ketolysis:** Your body turns to ketolysis when glucose is low and it needs an alternative fuel source. When fasting or following a low-carbohydrate diet, your body starts breaking down stored fat into ketone bodies, which can be used by tissues like the brain, heart, and muscles for energy.

- **Glycogenolysis:** Glycogenolysis is the breakdown of glycogen, the stored form of glucose, into glucose molecules. It's like tapping into a quick-access energy reserve. The body primarily uses glycogenolysis during short bursts of energy demand, such as intense exercise, or to maintain blood glucose levels between meals. Glycogen stores are limited, however, and can become depleted fairly quickly, especially during prolonged physical activity or fasting.

- **Gluconeogenesis:** Your cells can make new glucose from non-carbohydrate sources, including amino acids (from proteins) and glycerol (from fats). The body uses gluconeogenesis to keep blood glucose levels stable for essential functions, even when carbohydrate intake is low, as during prolonged fasting or starvation. This is important for tissues that can't use ketones, like red blood cells and certain parts of the kidney.

When you put all these processes together, as in the following illustration, it's very clear that making energy is a major priority for your body. There are many different ways the cells and mitochondria generate power, using multiple fuel sources.[116] Our job is to provide the fuel and other resources, including oxygen, to maximize cellular energy production. Our cells will take it from there.

How our cells use food to generate power

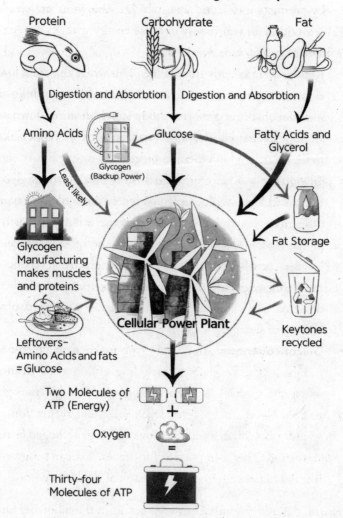

Protein   Carbohydrate   Fat

Digestion and Absorbtion   Digestion and Absorbtion

Amino Acids   Glucose   Fatty Acids and
                                       Glycerol

Glycogen
(Backup Power)

Least likely

Glycogen
Manufacturing
makes muscles
and proteins

Fat Storage

Cellular Power Plant

Leftovers–
Amino Acids and fats
= Glucose

Keytones
recycled

Two Molecules of
ATP (Energy)

+

Oxygen

=

Thirty-four
Molecules of ATP

Signals: Running Twenty-Four Seven

The fire Element is the driving force behind cellular energy creation and other biochemical reactions that keep you alive. Without it, life as we know it would cease to exist. However, fire has also been the most misunderstood of the classical elements. Traditional healers didn't know exactly what this fire was, but modern Western medicine has figured it out. Sophisticated machinery now exists to measure the fire—or, in technical terms, the electrical activity—in your body, including an EKG machine for your heart and an EEG machine for your brain.

This electrical activity is one of the ways cells signal each other, and those cell signals run the complex processes of life. When cells can "talk" to each other with signals, they thrive in rich, interdependent communities, where the health and function of one supports the vitality of others. Fire sustains the conversations between cells that are fundamental to life's continuity and harmony. In these interconnected communities, chemistry meets communication, proving that sometimes the smallest things can wield the most power. Within the cell, molecules exchange crucial information that determine everything from growth and healing to defense and reproduction. This communication is vital; without it, cells wouldn't know when to divide, when to fight off invaders, or when to repair damaged tissue so you can stay well.

As you may remember, cells communicate in four different ways:

Cell Signals

Direct Signals

Chemical Signals

Electrical Signals

Mechanical Signals

+ **Direct Signals:** Cells can communicate through direct contact. Some cells have structures on their surface that allow them to physically interact with neighboring cells. This direct contact can transmit signals between cells and facilitate processes like cell growth, differentiation, and movement.

+ **Chemical Signals:** When one cell wants to send a message to another cell, it releases special molecules called signaling molecules into its surroundings. These molecules can travel across short distances to nearby cells or through the bloodstream to reach cells in other parts of the body. When the signaling molecules reach the target cell, they bind to specific receptors, which triggers a response such as activating certain genes. This starts a metabolic process, which causes the cell to change its behavior.

+ **Electrical Signals:** In certain tissues, such as nerve cells, electrical impulses travel along specialized structures called axons to transmit information from one cell to another.

+ **Mechanical Signals:** Physical forces like stretching or compression can also act as signals to cells. For example, when cells experience mechanical stress, they can release signaling molecules that inform neighboring cells to adapt to the changes in their environment. This plays a crucial role in tissue development and wound healing.

When cell signals are working well, your body can energize, organize, and protect itself. As an example, let's take the sympathetic nervous system—your body's emergency alert system, which kicks into action when you encounter a threat. Whether it's a physical threat like a car speeding toward you or a psychological stressor like a deadline, cell signals get right to work. Let's walk through what this looks like:

1. Your brain identifies a threat and sends signals to the sympathetic nervous system.

2. This signal activates a cascade of signals throughout your body, preparing you to either fight the threat or flee from it. One key signaling molecule is adrenaline. Adrenaline is released from the adrenal

glands (which you learned about in chapter 1) into the bloodstream, signaling various target tissues and organs to prepare for action.

3. The adrenaline triggers a series of rapid and coordinated changes in your body.

4. Heart rate and blood pressure increase to deliver more oxygen and nutrients to your muscles and organs.

5. Your airways open wider to get more oxygen for energy production.

6. Your pupils dilate to enhance vision.

7. Nonessential bodily functions, like digestion and immune responses, are turned off.

These physiological changes prepare the body for rapid and quick action, allowing you to respond to a threat in a matter of seconds.

Cell signals are also key in healing after an injury. Consider what happens when you get a cut on your skin. The injury kicks off a dramatic, highly coordinated emergency response in the cells in the area. Let's take a closer look:

1. Blood clotting: The moment the skin is breached, injured blood vessels respond by mechanically squeezing to reduce blood loss. Circulating platelets in the bloodstream stick to the injury site, clumping together to form a clot. This clot acts as a temporary barrier against invaders, like bacteria, and as scaffolding for the needed upcoming repair work.

2. Inflammation: The cells damaged by the cut release chemicals, including cytokines and chemokines. These signals rapidly recruit immune cells like neutrophils and macrophages to the site, which begin cleaning up debris and warding off infections, leading to sore, red inflammation.

3. Rebuilding: At the same time, these immune cells and injured tissues release growth factors which direct the rebuilding, prompting nearby uninjured cells to grow and migrate to the wound site. The cut also disrupts the electrical current that your body maintains across the surface of your skin, and this disruption generates weak

electrical currents which act like traffic signals at an intersection, guiding cells to where they are most needed.

4. Healing: As new cells arrive and infrastructure is rebuilt, direct cell-to-cell signals ensure that the repair is seamless and intact. Once the cut is securely closed and the immediate threat has passed, the chemical signals change, telling immune cells to wind down the response and clean up any leftover garbage. All this to heal one cut! Your body's abilities are truly miraculous.

When Cell Signaling Goes Wrong

Cell signaling can also go seriously wrong. If cell signals malfunction, the immune system not only defends your body against disease and infection, but also mistakenly attacks healthy cells, tissues, and organs, leading to autoimmune disease. Autoimmune disease affects as many as fifty million people in the U.S., making it the third-most common disease category after cancer and heart disease. These attacks lead to inflammation and damage in different parts of the body, depending on the specific condition. For example, rheumatoid arthritis causes damage to the joints, while multiple sclerosis damages the nerves, additionally leaving those areas low in energy and unprotected from other threats. Autoimmune diseases can have a significant impact on a person's quality of life, leading to chronic symptoms, disability, and in some cases, life-threatening complications.[117]

What can interfere with cell signaling and lead to diseases like autoimmune disease? While there are many internal and external factors that can negatively affect these cell functions, two that are particularly impactful in our twenty-first-century world are chemical exposures and electromagnetic fields (EMFs).

Chemicals, Electromagnetic Frequencies, and Cell Signals

Certain environmental pollutants, termed "endocrine-disrupting chemicals," can interfere with signaling pathways by mimicking or blocking the action of your body's own hormones and other signaling molecules. These chemicals include:

✦ BPAs in plastics
✦ Phthalates and parabens in personal care products
✦ Per- and polyfluoroalkyl substances (PFAS) in nonstick cookware
✦ Glyphosate in herbicides used for agriculture

Exposure to these pollutants has been linked to reproductive and developmental abnormalities, metabolic disorders, and cancer.[118]

Studies also show that exposure to EMFs, such as those emitted by mobile phones or Wi-Fi routers, can change cellular signaling, impacting various cellular processes, including nerve function, muscle contraction, and gene expression. Compared with those that didn't use a mobile phone, users were found to be at higher risk for tumors, eye diseases, headaches, and mental health disorders.[119] Minimizing exposure to both chemicals and EMFs will maintain the efficacy of your cells' signals.

Modifying Cellular Signals with Caffeine

When interfered with, your cellular signals can be strengthened, muffled, or even turned off completely. Many medications, remedies, and even foods intentionally work to do just that.

Caffeine is one of those foods. A survey of thirty-seven thousand people found that 85 percent of the U.S. population consumes at least one caffeinated beverage per day.[120] Ever wondered why people reach for that cup of coffee or tea when they need a pick-me-up? Well, let's dive into the cell science behind that caffeine buzz.

Your brain releases a chemical signal called adenosine. As it gets later in the day, adenosine levels slowly rise, signaling to your brain that it's time to wind down and get sleepy. You can disrupt this sleepy signal with caffeine. Caffeine's structure is very similar to adenosine, which allows it to sneak in and bind to brain cells in adenosine's place, preventing the drowsy response from starting. In fact, instead of drowsiness, caffeine flips the switch for alertness. Neurons fire up, releasing a flood of feel-good neurotransmitters like dopamine and norepinephrine. Suddenly, you're not just awake; you're buzzing with energy, laser-focused, ready to tackle whatever the day throws your way.

This sounds like it could be an answer to society's low energy problem, but it's not. While caffeine can provide a temporary feeling of energy being boosted, consuming too much can lead to effects you don't want, like jitteriness, insomnia, a post-caffeine energy crash, and dependence. But the biggest problem with caffeine is that it doesn't give your cells what they actually need: energy! And because you feel more energized after having caffeine, you continue to push your body, using up even more of its dwindling energy reserves. In effect, caffeine turns off your body's warning signs that it needs something, and allows you to burn through your energy reserves, leaving little left for other essential functions.

Covering up Cell Signals

Feeling the need to reach for a cup of coffee or an energy drink is a symptom of low cellular energy. Your internal cellular systems run best on high-power mode, and symptoms like feeling sluggish, tired, or exhausted are indicators that you need to pay attention to rather than cover up with caffeine. Now, I know I'm not going to win any popularity contests telling people to give up their caffeine! In all likelihood, you're one of the 85 percent of people who use caffeine daily to deal with low cellular energy. What other options do you have?

But remember, cellular energy is all about fire. You can increase that fire in your cells each morning in a few simple-to-implement ways:

+ Exercise! A fifteen-minute session of interval training will boost mitochondrial energy production and make it more efficient.
+ Stick to complex carbohydrates like fruits and vegetables for your morning meal. Complex carbs provide a steadier supply of fuel than quick-burning simple carbohydrates like bagels or cold cereal and

milk. Instead of these foods, consider trying an egg scramble with mushrooms or zucchini.

✦ Take a cold shower. Cold exposure can increase the number and activity of mitochondria in the cells, as well as expand the blood vessels carrying oxygenated blood so those mitochondria get more oxygen for energy production.[121]

Caffeine isn't the only common way to cover up your cells' signals. If you have a splitting headache, you can take a pain reliever, and the headache pain usually goes away. That pill didn't make you healthy or address the cause of the headache; it simply turned off the signal that something was wrong. If you have a congested nose, you can take a decongestant and your nasal passages clear. Again, that decongestant didn't make the cold or allergy go away or fix anything in your sinuses; it just covered up the signal for a while. Unfortunately, people have been taught to think that this is enough or all the relief anyone can hope for. But caffeine, pain relievers, and decongestants are all smoke screens. The warning signs they block out are a key part of the cell talk that is going on constantly in your body.

Cell Signals Preserve Life

Sometimes it's dangerous to turn off cell signals. These signals literally preserve your life. Cellular signaling is the language your body uses, and you can learn to translate this language. My grandfather, John, was a cardiologist and learned to translate the cell signals that operate the heart. He had spent his career listening to and learning the rhythms of other people's hearts. Yet when it came to the irregular beats of his own, he turned a deaf ear. He dismissed an occasional skipped beat as nothing more than a symptom of his age. A passionate runner, he would pound the pavement in the early hours before dawn, getting his miles in before heading to the office or hospital. His dedication to running wasn't just for the love of the sport; it was his way of strengthening his own body, and he often prescribed running and exercise to his patients long before it was common practice to do so.

Over the years, his heart had grown strong, capable of pumping very efficiently, thanks in part to his consistent training. One afternoon like any other, John laced up his running shoes and set out for a seven-mile run over his lunch break. As he picked up his pace, he felt his heart skip beats, the signal failures he'd grown accustomed to ignoring. This time, however, the skip was followed by a sudden darkness. His heart had stopped. He collapsed face-first onto the side of the road, hitting the ground with a jarring impact. Miraculously, the fall that brought him down also jolted his heart back to action. Strong from years of running, John's heart restarted. He regained consciousness with a bloody nose and skinned knees and elbows, and he quickly realized what had happened. He knew too much, had seen too much, and had ignored it too long. He needed a pacemaker.

A pacemaker, a small electrical device implanted under the skin of the chest, is designed to restore the natural rhythm and signals of the heart. It works by sending electrical impulses to the heart to ensure it beats regularly, compensating for any irregularities or disturbances in the heart's own electrical cell signaling. For John, whose heart had the strength but not the proper signaling to function well, the pacemaker would maintain the cell signals that kept him alive. With the pacemaker in place, John felt a new sense of security. He returned to running and ran competitively into his late seventies.

Signals and Signs

Each signal contributes to a finely balanced ecosystem within the body, and when these signals go awry, it can lead to diseases like cancer, where cells grow uncontrollably, or diabetes, where the signal to regulate blood sugar is ignored. Thankfully, the body has ways of alerting us when things aren't working right. My patient, Natalie, a vibrant twenty-two-year-old college student, was noticing some troubling signs but didn't know what they meant. She had started to feel increasingly tired but attributed it to her hectic schedule, as she juggled classes, part-time work, and social activities. She had sore gums, even though she took meticulous care of her teeth, and her tongue was always red and tender. The fatigue persisted, her sore gums started to bleed, and she began noticing other troubling symptoms. While studying in the library one day, Natalie suddenly felt lightheaded and dizzy. She reached for her water bottle, hoping hydration would help, but the dizziness continued.

Concerned, her mom recommended she visit my office. My team checked her gums, and seeing no signs of gum disease, we knew it was time to check her blood sugar levels. We sent her to the clinic on campus where she could be seen that day. A nurse checked her vital signs and ran a series of tests, including a blood sugar measurement. When the results came back, the nurse's expression was serious. Natalie's blood sugar levels were dangerously high. Confused and frightened, Natalie was referred to a specialist. After further testing, she received a diagnosis that shocked her: type 1 diabetes. It explained her fatigue, bleeding gums, frequent thirst, and unexplained weight loss over the past few months. Natalie had been living with undiagnosed diabetes, unaware of how much of a toll it was taking on her body.

Though she was devastated, Natalie was lucky to have advanced diabetes treatments available to her. In the early twentieth century, diabetes was a poorly understood and often fatal disease. Patients with diabetes experienced extreme thirst, frequent urination, weight loss, and sometimes even coma or death. Scientists knew the pancreas had a role to play in this disease, as autopsies of diabetic patients often showed problems in this organ, but exactly how the disease worked was a mystery.

In 1921, a breakthrough occurred. A team of researchers at the University of Toronto, led by Dr. Frederick Banting and his assistant Charles Best, discovered that a hormone called insulin, extracted from the pancreas of healthy dogs, could be injected into diabetic dogs to stabilize their blood sugar levels. This discovery revolutionized the treatment of diabetes and has saved countless lives. It also highlighted how cell signaling is at the center of blood sugar balance in the body.

How does it work? Let's see the signaling in action!

+ When you eat a meal that contains glucose or sugar, the sugar enters your bloodstream.
+ This rise in blood sugar levels triggers the pancreas to release insulin, a signaling molecule produced there, into the bloodstream.
+ This finely tuned signaling molecule then binds to receptors on the surface of cells that need glucose, such as muscle, fat, and liver cells.
+ The insulin binding initiates a cascade of signaling and activity inside the cells, telling their cellular machinery to allow glucose to enter the cell from the bloodstream.

In people with diabetes, either the pancreas does not produce enough insulin (type 1 diabetes), or the body's cells become resistant to the effects of insulin, ignoring the signal and failing to initiate the process to bring glucose in (type 2 diabetes). In both cases, the cellular signaling pathways controlled by insulin are affected, resulting in too much sugar left in the bloodstream. These elevated blood sugar levels lead to the serious symptoms associated with diabetes.

The discovery of insulin and its signaling pathways not only completely changed the treatment of diabetes—but also provided new insight into the importance of cell signaling in maintaining overall health. It highlighted the intricate communication between cells and the essential role this communication plays in keeping your cells running.

How to Interpret Cell Signals

Natalie wasn't happy about her diabetes diagnosis, but she found ways to help her cells communicate with one another again. She had to learn how to monitor her blood sugar levels, administer insulin injections, and make changes to her diet and lifestyle. But by supporting her cells, she was able to gradually adapt to her new reality and find a way to be well. In Natalie's cells and yours, the communication between cells is essential for coordinating cell growth, wound healing, nutrient uptake and storage, hormone messaging, the immune system, responses to the environment, and more. It's a complex conversation happening at the microscopic level, ensuring that the body functions harmoniously as a whole.

Cell signaling is how your cells communicate, and nothing happens, good or bad, in the cell without this signal or instruction. When the signaling works as designed, your cells can keep themselves healthy. When the signaling slows or stops, or when you cover it up with medications, your cells, and you, get sick and age. The Cell Well model is the "Google Translate" that will help you interpret your cells' language of signals. When all four divisions in the cell are working properly to support this cellular communication, you can create limitless energy. And when you provide your cells with more energy, you turn up the wellness in your life.

Chapter 5
Keyhole Concepts

- ✦ When your cells have energy, they provide you with energy. Once you understand that relationship, you can make choices that will help you provide your cells with the energy they need.
- ✦ Your daily food choices supply the fuel that your body's mitochondria require to continue to function normally. This fuel brings energy potential to the cells and determines how much energy they can generate.
- ✦ Your cells' mitochondria only work when they are provided with the correct fuel. If you provide poor quality fuel that has little "energy potential" in it, your cells' mitochondria won't have optimal output.
- ✦ Signaling, or "cell talk," is how your cells communicate. When the signaling works as designed, your cells can keep themselves healthy. When the signaling slows or stops, your cells, and you, get sick and age.
- ✦ Cellular communication also allows your cellular communities to collectively solve problems. The cells that are the best at communicating, adapting, and problem-solving are the ones that survive.

CHAPTER 6

Plants

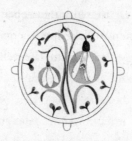

Plants, and the earth that supports them, provide the compounds that deliver necessary and restorative nutrients to your body and cells. Plants are both food and medicine and should form the foundation of both your diet and medicine kit. Together, we will explore the history and science of the diet and nutrition recommendations you may be familiar with today. We'll also learn about why processed foods have become such a prominent part of the food supply, and why these foods don't feed your cells and body what they need. You will also learn what marketing claims and labels on processed foods really mean, and how to navigate the trending concerns about plant compounds like lectins and phytates.

Before modern medicine, people learned about plants as food and medicine from their grandmothers and other elders in their community.

Blueberries are native to North America and have been consumed by Indigenous peoples for thousands of years. They gathered and used these delicious berries because their people always had, and whenever they ate blueberries, the fruit soothed the elders' arthritis, helped the entire tribe fend off seasonal illnesses, and kept their bowels moving. It helped them stay well.

Science can now tell us which compounds found in blueberries help our cells stay well. Blueberries are packed with vitamins, minerals, antioxidants, and phytochemicals, most notably vitamin C, vitamin K, manganese, fiber, and the flavonoids that give them their recognizable deep purple color. Blueberries are known to help combat oxidative stress, a condition that occurs when there are too many unstable, damaging molecules called free radicals in the body and not enough antioxidants to get rid of them. The high levels of antioxidants in blueberries, particularly flavonoids like anthocyanins, neutralize inflammation, relax blood vessels (leading to lower blood pressure), and improve cholesterol levels, which together lead to a reduced risk of heart disease, cancer, and stroke. Additionally, the fiber in the berries, along with those abundant antioxidants, help to improve memory and mood, eye health, and blood sugar regulation.

Blueberries check all the Cell Well boxes:

+ **Supply:** These tasty berries supply your body with essential vitamins, minerals, and more.
+ **Support:** Support for many cellular systems, including the digestive and cardiovascular systems, come from their fiber and flavonoids.
+ **Secure:** They secure the cell against free radical damage and inflammation with their protective antioxidants.
+ **Signal:** They improve signaling in far-reaching systems, boosting blood sugar regulation as well as mood and memory.

Nutrition Science and the Birth
of the Supplement Industry

Nutrition science, the field of study focused on understanding how food and nutrition impact human health and disease, is a young science. It wasn't until the early 1900s that scientists made big discoveries about essential vitamins and minerals. They found that certain illnesses, like scurvy and beriberi, were caused by not having enough of certain important nutrients.[122] One scientist, Casimir Funk, coined the term "vitamin" in a study of these diseases.[123] By the middle of the century, scientists had identified and made synthetic versions of all the major vitamins, and single-vitamin supplements, focused on a specific deficiency, became available. This is when the vitamin supplement industry took off.

At the same time, manufacturers started adding extra nutrients to staple foods like salt and flour.[124] This helped reduce conditions caused by vitamin and mineral deficiencies, like goiters and rickets. Interestingly, all this happened during the Great Depression and World War II, when worries about food access were widespread, and preventing nutrient deficiencies was very important. In fact, the first Recommended Dietary Allowances were created in 1941 to help people get enough nutrients during wartime.[125]

Over the next couple of decades, better economic conditions and fortified staple foods drastically reduced malnutrition and vitamin deficiencies in wealthier countries. But as this progress continued, attention turned to a new challenge: diet-related diseases. Researchers explored the links between fat and sugar intake and health issues like heart disease.[126] Initially, fat was blamed, leading to widespread adoption of low-fat diets, though some nutritionists argued that the evidence wasn't strong enough to warrant such drastic measures. In less affluent nations, the focus remained on boosting calorie intake and consumption of essential nutrients. Food was seen as a delivery system for these vital elements, leading to innovations in the production of energy-dense staples like wheat and rice.

Through the 1970s, '80s, and '90s, countries and people grew wealthier, farming techniques improved, and nutritional deficiency diseases started to decline around the world. But while fewer people were suffering from diseases like scurvy and rickets, other diet-related diseases like obesity, diabetes, and certain cancers were on the rise. To tackle these new health challenges, governments began changing their nutrition guidelines. They focused less on preventing nutrient deficiencies and more on preventing chronic diseases. For example, the 1980 Dietary Guidelines for Americans advised people to eat less fat and sugar, and more fiber.[127] At the same time, there was a global effort to fight nutrient deficiencies in poorer countries.[128] Scientists found that giving people supplements like iron and vitamin A could prevent diseases like measles and blindness. They also started adding nutrients like iodine to salt to prevent conditions like goiters, an enlargement of the thyroid gland. The new focus was on making sure people got the right nutrients to stay healthy.

In recent years, there have been some big breakthroughs in this understanding of how our diets affect our health. Scientists have conducted large studies investigating how different foods and nutrients impact our bodies.[129] These studies have shown that just looking at one nutrient on its own isn't enough. For example, while we used to think cutting down on fat was the key to staying healthy, newer research suggests it's not that simple. Instead, it's about looking at the overall pattern of what we eat. We've learned that patterns of eating like the Mediterranean diet, which focuses on whole foods like fruits, veggies, and nuts, can be good for us. On the flip side, diets high in processed foods, sugar, and starch can do more harm than good.[130]

The Evolution of the Food Pyramid

The concept of a food pyramid dates to 1970s Sweden, but the United States didn't introduce its first version until 1992. This inaugural American food pyramid focused on grains as the base of the pyramid, followed by fruits and vegetables, then dairy and protein, with fats and sweets in a small section at the top. This pyramid was based on the prevailing understanding of nutrition at the time, which emphasized eating few fats and plenty of carbohydrates.

I lived through this low-fat era and ate my share of the famed fat-free and sugar-full SnackWell's cookies, incorrectly thinking that "low fat" meant that they were healthier. This simple pyramid faced widespread criticism from various quarters, including from nutritionists, health experts, and researchers. Some of their key targets of criticism included the pyramid's overemphasis on carbohydrates, its limited focus on fats and proteins, and its oversimplified dietary recommendations, which ignored nuances in nutrition and individual dietary needs. Fortunately, as scientific research evolved, so did the dietary guidelines.

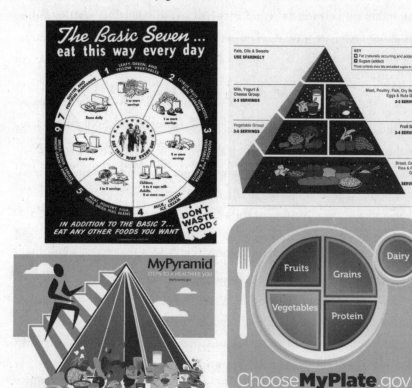

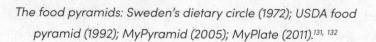

The food pyramids: Sweden's dietary circle (1972); USDA food pyramid (1992); MyPyramid (2005); MyPlate (2011).[131, 132]

In 2011, the United States Department of Agriculture (USDA) replaced the food pyramid with MyPlate, which offered a simpler visual representation of a balanced diet, featuring a plate divided into sections for fruits, vegetables, grains, and protein, with a side serving of dairy. It also emphasized the importance of quality over quantity, recommending whole grains, lean proteins, and healthy fats, while limiting added sugars and processed foods. Critics argue that the food pyramid, and even MyPlate to some extent, have been influenced by commercial agriculture interests. Was the emphasis on grains in the original food pyramid due to the lobbying power of the grain industry? Has the dairy industry had any influence on whether dairy-containing foods are on the "plate" or not?

What Makes a Food Healthy?

Studies support the claims that these guidelines are affected by more than just the health of consumers. After all, government policies heavily shape both the agricultural landscape and consumer dietary habits in the United States.[133] By subsidizing the production of specific crops, such as corn, wheat, and soy, the government influences their prevalence in the food supply. These highly subsidized crops are often the main "fillers" in processed foods, and since they're so ubiquitous, people eat far too many of them—no matter how many pyramids and plates the USDA designs.

This confusion between commercial interests and real nutrition became clear for me a few years ago when one of my team members, Bree, newly married and in her early twenties, was determined to get "healthier." In frustration, she told me she had been working to lose weight all through her teenage years. She thought of healthy foods as the "one-hundred-calorie" packs of her favorite processed snacks. Bree had even been skipping meals, trying crazy fad diets she saw on social media, and as a cheerleader, even overexercising. All her work had left her with no less weight—and much less energy. To add insult to injury, she got bloated when she ate the prepackaged, grain-filled snacks and had thinning hair, nails, and feelings of depression.

She knew there had to be a better way. Stretching her paycheck, she hired a trainer who taught her how to exercise more effectively and helped her redesign her snacks and meals with a focus on gaining energy rather than restricting calories. With a diet heavy on fresh produce (plants), Bree's body was finally getting the nourishment it needed to be healthy and full of energy, and let go of the weight it had held onto for years. She realized that eating fresh, unprocessed foods needed to become a way of life, not a diet. But why hadn't Bree's body not "figured this out" on its own earlier? According to the Cell Well model, shouldn't your cells know what they need and how to stay well?

Why Are You Hungry?

Your body has an amazing "hunger detector" that is managed through cell signaling. Because this detector is so much like a thermostat regulating your home's temperature, scientists have called it an "appestat," because it manages your appetite.[134] Located in the hypothalamus in the brain, the appestat is the control center for managing hunger and fullness. It constantly monitors various bodily indicators, including fat stores, gut hormones, blood sugar levels, and energy expenditure.[135]

Appestat – Nutrient Detector

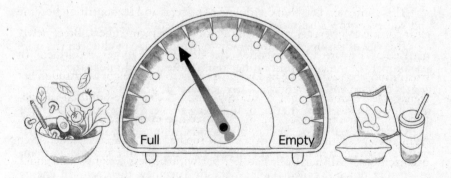

Do these sound familiar? They're some of the cell signals you learned about in chapter 5. They come from different parts of the body, and they help your brain decide when you're hungry or full. Hormones like ghrelin and leptin tell the brain to start or stop eating.[136] Cells in the gut send messages to the brain about how much food is in your system. Even sensory signals in your brain, like those that communicate the smell and sight of food, can trigger hunger. All these signals work together to help you know when to eat and when to stop, keeping your body in balance.

Bree struggled with having enough energy and losing weight because she wasn't feeding her body what it needed to function well. Although her body was "full" of calories from the processed foods and diet bars she was eating, what her body (and yours, too) really needed was nutrients. If you filled your car's gas tank with corn syrup, it would be full, but your car wouldn't go very far. Why? Because a car requires the proper type of fuel to run. So do you. Your tank can be full of processed, nutrient-deficient foods and you will still feel hungry because your cells need more fuel to create energy. They get that energy from foods with the right nutrients. This is why you can eat an entire bag of potato chips and still want more. Those potato chips did not deliver the nutrients necessary to turn your appestat off. Plants, in their whole, unprocessed form, are full of energy-giving nutrients that help regulate your systems and re-calibrate your appestat.

How Do Whole Foods Help?

Did you ever grow a bean seed in a cup in elementary school?

This rite of passage is a simple way to demonstrate to children the miracle of plants. The child pushes that resilient bean seed under the soil and douses the cup with water. The water activates all the nutrients and energy that has been stored in that seed, initiating the seed's growth, and within a few days, a seedling pushes out of the soil and into the sunlight. The first spindly growth stretches for the sun, activating the internal energy manufacturing process, called photosynthesis. Together, the chemical energy from the sun, and electrons and nutrients from the seed and soil, power up the plant, and it grows.

That bean plant and the beans it produces are filled with nutrients such as protein, dietary fiber, complex carbohydrates, vitamins (such as folate, vitamin B6, and vitamin K), minerals (such as iron, magnesium, potassium, and zinc), and phytonutrients (such as flavonoids and antioxidants): the things your cells need.

They are a whole, or real, food.

Processed foods often lack these essential nutrients or contain them in significantly reduced amounts due to refining, extraction, and other manufacturing processes. Additionally, processed foods may contain added sugars, unhealthy fats, and high levels of sodium, which can have detrimental effects on cellular health. Consuming nutrient-dense whole foods like beans in their whole form provides the necessary building blocks for cellular function and overall health that processed foods cannot adequately provide. When consumed like this, plants feed your bodies and cells.

In T. Colin Campbell's seminal book *Whole: Rethinking the Science of Nutrition*, Campbell takes a deep dive into the intricate relationship between food and nutrients. He argues that when it comes to plants, the whole is greater than the sum of its parts. Nutrients found in whole foods interact in complex ways within the body, creating synergistic effects that cannot be replicated if those nutrients are taken out of the food and eaten individually in processed foods or supplements.

For example, he explains that eating an apple gives your body far more than just the vitamins, minerals, fiber, and phytochemicals that it is made of. While all those individual components play important roles in nutrition, they interact with each other in ways that just can't be reproduced outside of the whole fruit. For instance, when you isolate the vitamin C from an apple and take it as a supplement, it doesn't give the same health benefits for your cells and body as you would get if you snacked on the whole apple. The vitamin C in the apple interacts with other compounds, such as fiber and antioxidants, which help your body absorb and use the vitamin C. The fiber in the apple also helps regulate digestion, promote gut health, and slows down absorption of the sugars in the gut—all benefits you wouldn't get if you just took a fiber pill.

Nutrients in an Apple

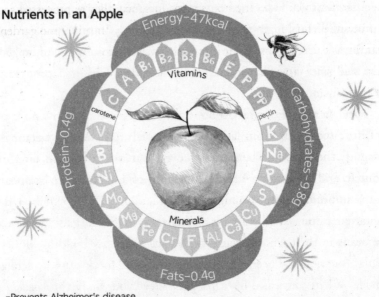

-Prevents Alzheimer's disease
-Reduces the risk of pancreatic and breast cancer
-Relieves swelling
-Protects against formation of gallstones
-Reduces fluctuation in blood sugar
-Reduces the incidence of respiratory diseases(including asthma)
-Improves digestion
-Cleanses the liver
-Reduces cholesterol
-Strengthens the immune system

Whole plants are complex matrices of nutrients and bioactive compounds that work together to fuel cell energy and promote health. To truly harness these powers and benefits, you need to eat food that is as close to its natural state as possible.[137]

Processed Versus Whole Foods

Since processed foods became popular in the twentieth century, the Western diet has shifted more and more toward ready-to-eat meals. These convenient meals cater to the modern on-the-go lifestyle, and may even cost less, but they can negatively affect your health and energy.

To make this clearer, let's talk about what "processing" really means. Almost all foods undergo some level of processing, even if it's just to make them shelf-stable. Take dried beans, for instance; they're processed so they can be stored for longer periods without spoiling. In my home garden one year, I was excited to grow the kind of beans you dry and use to make bean soup and other tasty bean dishes. I planned to harvest, dry, and store them for the winter.

After they were done growing, I put all the bean pods in a plastic bag, sealed it, and didn't think about it for a few weeks. When I returned to that bag, the pods and beans were covered in mold. I hadn't dried them properly, and the improper handling led me to lose my entire bean harvest that year. Some handling and processing are necessary for foods, and this processing doesn't inherently make them unhealthy. Researchers have designated four categories of processing for foods:[138]

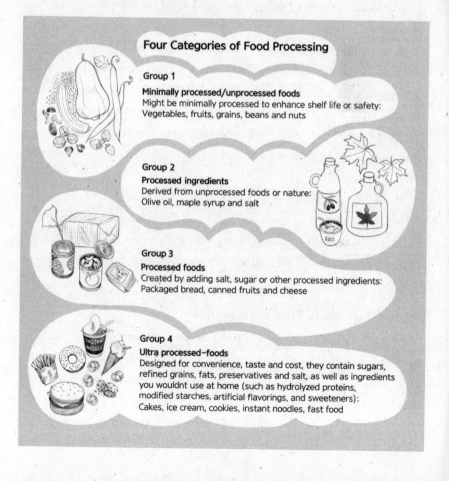

Four Categories of Food Processing

Group 1

Minimally processed/unprocessed foods
Might be minimally processed to enhance shelf life or safety:
Vegetables, fruits, grains, beans and nuts

Group 2
Processed ingredients
Derived from unprocessed foods or nature:
Olive oil, maple syrup and salt

Group 3
Processed foods
Created by adding salt, sugar or other processed ingredients:
Packaged bread, canned fruits and cheese

Group 4
Ultra processed-foods
Designed for convenience, taste and cost, they contain sugars, refined grains, fats, preservatives and salt, as well as ingredients you wouldnt use at home (such as hydrolyzed proteins, modified starches, artificial flavorings, and sweeteners):
Cakes, ice cream, cookies, instant noodles, fast food

Plants fall into the first two categories. This category typically provides the most nutrients and energy for your cells and body. For example, one cup of red bell peppers, kiwi fruit, or orange slices contains more than 100 percent of the amount of vitamin C you're recommended to consume daily.[139] That vitamin C is part of the support team for your cells, managing growth and repair of tissues, building collagen, skin, cartilage, tendons, ligaments, and blood vessels. It is also needed for healing wounds and repairing and maintaining bones and teeth.[140] Eat your peppers, kiwi, and oranges! Equally impressively, a single Brazil nut provides all the selenium you need for an entire day. Selenium helps to make DNA and protects the cell against cell damage and infections.[141] One Brazil nut a day is a tasty, simple prescription for healthier cells.

Minimally processed foods also avoid the problems that come with high levels of sugar. If you feed your body sugary, processed food, your blood sugar spikes, depleting your insulin reserves and leading to an energy crash. Studies show that continually eating these processed, sugary foods affects your cells' ability to respond to insulin signals. Like the story of the boy who cried wolf, when your cells are constantly being told to open the gates and let sugar in, they eventually stop listening. This elevates the risk of developing obesity, insulin resistance, type 2 diabetes, fatty liver disease, and heart disease.[142]

You may be thinking, what about the sugar in fruit? Fruits contain lots of fiber, and the type of sugar found in fruit, called fructose, is bound to the fiber, which slows its absorption in the gut and minimizes the impact on your cells' insulin.[143] We will learn more about this later in the chapter.

Processed Foods Aren't Nourishing

Processed foods, including white flour baked goods, pasta, salad oil, mayonnaise, doughnuts, cookies, rice cakes, breakfast bars, chips, soda, candy, or popcorn, lack significant nutrients to supply your cells with what they need.

Dr. Joel Fuhrman, a whole foods champion, introduced a new approach to eating called the "nutritarian diet." This eating plan is designed to maximize the amount of nutrients you get in your diet and can deliver to your cells. Specifically, Dr. Fuhrman suggests that at least 90 percent of your daily caloric intake should come from plant foods, such as fruits, vegetables, legumes, nuts, and seeds. The remaining 10 percent can include animal products or processed foods, but these should be consumed in moderation. In the nutritarian diet, the focus is on maximizing the intake of nutrient-dense plant foods to promote optimal health and longevity.[144]

Living Well with Dr. Michelle doesn't prescribe any diet plan over another, but this diet serves as a good example of one way eating for wellness can look. We can compare this nutrient-based approach to the common fare in the Standard American Diet, where over 55 percent of its calories come from processed foods, 33 percent from animal products, and a mere 10 percent from fresh produce (including French fries and ketchup). Full of chemicals and synthetic additives, corn syrup, sugar, artificial sweeteners, salt, and coloring agents, this diet contains a lot of calories and tastes great, but offers nothing to cells, making it difficult to stay well.

How Your Cells Use Nutrients

Now that you know why a balanced diet rich in a variety of real, whole foods and nutrient-dense plants are so essential for cell health, let's talk about how your cells use them.

Nutrients that SUPPLY the Cells

Carbohydrates and Fats Make Energy (ATP)

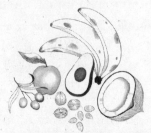

Come from: rice, potatoes, wheat,
apples, bananas, avocado, coconut,
olives, almonds, and, walnuts

Vitamins and Minerals Build DNA and RNA

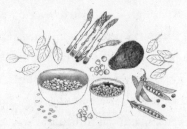

Come from: spinach, asparagus,
broccoli, avocado, lentils, chickpeas,
black beans, and, peas

✦ **Produce Energy:** Carbohydrates and fats are broken down in the mitochondria during cellular metabolism to make energy in the form of ATP to fuel the cells. (Flip back to chapter 5 to see this explained in detail.)

✦ **Make DNA and RNA:** Micronutrients like folate, vitamin B6, vitamin B12, zinc, magnesium, and iron are the architects and repair teams of our genetic material. Folate and B12 lay down the foundation of DNA, ensuring that the blueprint of life is accurately copied and passed on. Vitamin B6 oversees and regulates the chemical reactions that are essential for DNA construction and repair. Zinc and magnesium are vital for the function of enzymes that stitch together and mend DNA strands. Iron, meanwhile, supplies the raw materials needed to construct these DNA building blocks.[145]

Nutrients that SUPPORT the Cells

Proteins and Fats Build Cells

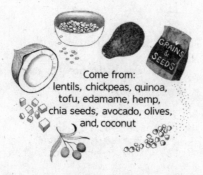

Come from:
lentils, chickpeas, quinoa,
tofu, edamame, hemp,
chia seeds, avocado, olives,
and, coconut

Enzymes (Special Proteins) Speed Up Cell Activity

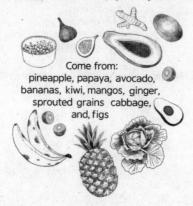

Come from:
pineapple, papaya, avocado,
bananas, kiwi, mangos, ginger,
sprouted grains cabbage,
and, figs

✦ **Give Cells Structure:** Proteins and fats are the essential to our cells. Proteins are like the bricks and mortar, and construct vital components such as the nucleus, where genetic information is housed, and the mitochondria, the powerhouse that directs energy production. Meanwhile, fats form the cell membrane, the protective barrier that surrounds each cell, controlling what enters and exits the cell.[146]

✦ **Help with Cellular Reactions:** Enzymes are specialized proteins that speed up the countless chemical reactions that sustain life. Without them, even the simplest processes, like digesting food or repairing DNA, would take ages to complete. What makes enzymes truly fascinating is their ability to adapt and respond to their environment. Enzymes ensure that our bodies can react swiftly and efficiently to whatever challenges come their way, making them indispensable to life as we know it.[147]

Nutrients that SECURE the Cells

Antioxidants Protect from Damage

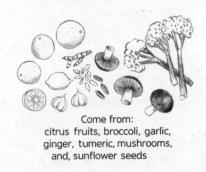

Come from:
citrus fruits, broccoli, garlic,
ginger, tumeric, mushrooms,
and, sunflower seeds

Vitamins and Minerals Build the Immune System

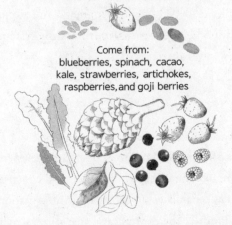

Come from:
blueberries, spinach, cacao,
kale, strawberries, artichokes,
raspberries, and goji berries

✦ **Protect the Cell:** Antioxidants in plants act as nature's defense system, protecting cells from the relentless attack of free radicals—unstable molecules that can cause significant damage or oxidative stress in the body. Free radicals can lead to the deterioration of cells, contributing to aging and the development of various diseases, including cancer and heart disease. Antioxidants can neutralize them because they are able to donate a stabilizing electron without becoming unstable themselves. Examples of antioxidants include anthocyanins in blueberries, flavonoids in green tea, and vitamin C in citrus fruits.[148]

✦ **Build Immune Function:** Nutrients like vitamins A, C, and D, along with minerals such as zinc and selenium, arm your immune system against invaders. Vitamin A maintains the integrity of your skin and mucous membranes—your body's first line of defense against pathogens. Vitamin C stimulates the production of white blood cells and enhances their ability to protect the body. Vitamin D ensures that your body can respond appropriately to various threats without going overboard. Zinc is vital for the development and function of immune cells, and selenium, a powerful antioxidant, works to prevent cellular damage and supports the production of antibodies, enhancing your immune system's ability to fight off viruses and bacteria.[149]

Nutrients that SIGNAL the Cells

Indirect Antioxidants Detox the Cells

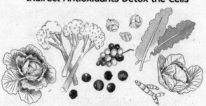

Come from:
broccoli, brussels sprouts,
kale, cauliflower, cabbage,
tumeric, red grapes, and, blueberries

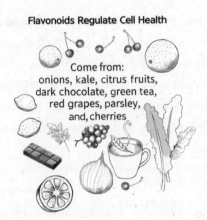

Flavonoids Regulate Cell Health

Come from:
onions, kale, citrus fruits,
dark chocolate, green tea,
red grapes, parsley,
and, cherries

✦ **Detoxify the Body and Cells:** Indirect antioxidants, like sulfora-phane, curcumin, and resveratrol, are like the body's own elite detox squad, supercharging your natural defenses to keep your cells clean and functioning at their best. It's like having a built-in cleanup crew that's always on duty, ensuring your body stays clear of toxins and free radicals.[150] But the magic doesn't stop there—these antioxidants are also the best allies your liver could ask for. Indirect antioxidants like sulforaphane give the liver a helping hand by boosting the activity of its detoxifying enzymes, making the entire process more efficient.

✦ **Regulate Cell Health:** Flavonoids, the colorful compounds found in many fruits and vegetables, play a dynamic role in cell signaling, acting as molecular messengers that can influence a wide range of biological processes. When you consume foods rich in flavonoids, like berries, apples, or onions, these compounds interact with various signaling pathways in your cells, influencing cell growth, dif-ferentiation, and survival. These versatile compounds also play a crucial role in regulating inflammation and oxidative stress—two processes that, when uncontrolled, can lead to chronic diseases.[151]

The benefits of long-beloved foods like blueberries are clear, and no one debates their value in your diet. However, if you look at a list of other foods your ancestors gathered, cultivated, and filled their bowls with, you'll find many plant foods that are heavily debated in today's online "nutrition wars."

Conflicting studies, clickbait claims, and passionate rhetoric often fuel the skirmishes, as different camps vie for influence over public opinion and consumer choices in the ever-evolving landscape of nutrition and wellness.[152] How can you and I sort through this deluge of information to find what will help you and your cells be well? Could some compounds in plants be harmful? You might have seen some of these clickbait statements or others like them:

✦ "Are Lectins Poisoning Your Plate?"
✦ "Think Your Salad Is Safe? Think Again: The Hidden Dangers of Oxalates Revealed"
✦ "The Whole Truth About Whole Foods: Health Risks Dietitians Won't Tell You"
✦ "Do You Know What Your Organic Labels Are Hiding?"
✦ "Could Your Whole Foods Diet be a Recipe for Disaster?"

These statements often leave out the "rest of the story."

Let's tackle some common controversies about plants and nutrition. Eating and getting the nutrients your cells need should not be difficult! So we will walk through the latest research to clear up what's hype and what's proven and give you the keys to understand plants and the amazing benefits they provide.

Is Grain Still the Staff of Life?

For thousands of years, wheat and other grains have been a cornerstone of the global food supply. Today, wheat alone provides around one-fifth of the world's calories and protein.[153] In 2023, 787 million tons of wheat were produced globally, a volume comparable to the combined weight of over two thousand Empire State Buildings. Wheat and other grains literally feed the world.[154]

Bread made from wheat, rye, or other grains has long been a diet staple in many different cultures. The fact that a phrase like "Give us this day our daily bread" even appears in prayers just goes to show how important grains have been to civilizations throughout history. However, in recent years, grain's image has been tarnished, especially with the rise of criticism against gluten. I myself have eaten a largely gluten-free diet for over five years. While gluten-free eating is essential for those with celiac disease or non-celiac gluten sensitivity, many others have adopted it out of a fear that gluten may be harmful.

Is this fear warranted? Wheat and other grains have also come under scrutiny because of their most common form in the modern diet: refined grain products. These processed "carbs," often packed with added sugars and chemicals, are frequently associated with weight gain, inflammation, and other chronic health issues. This has led to a broader debate over whether wheat is truly beneficial to modern consumers or if it is a major contributor to health problems like obesity and chronic disease.[155]

The key to understanding this discussion lies in differentiating between whole, minimally processed grains and the refined grain products that dominate many diets today. Whole grains can offer significant health benefits, whereas refined grains are often linked to negative health outcomes.[156] For example:

+ A 2016 analysis of nearly eight hundred thousand people in the U.S. revealed a strong correlation between eating more whole grains and a reduced risk of disease, including cardiovascular disease and cancer. The researchers recommended at least three servings of whole grains per day to support long-term health and longevity.[157]

+ A 2022 Harvard Medical School analysis of nearly two hundred thousand people, followed for an average of over twenty-five years, reported that more whole grain intake was associated with lower heart disease risk.[158]

+ A 2018 article concluded that people who eat two to three servings of whole grains per day reduce their risk of developing type 2 diabetes by 21–32 percent.[159]

+ A 2016 study from Imperial College London discovered that whole grains could also protect against cancer. People who ate three or more servings per day were 15 percent less likely to develop cancer than those who ate lower amounts of whole grains.[160]

✦ A 2023 clinical trial, which for eight years followed almost three thousand people who had or were at risk for arthritis, found that people who ate more whole grains had a lower chance of developing severe arthritis.

✦ Another 2023 study showed that whole grains and their accompanying dietary fiber can help support a beneficial gut microbiome, with some of the healthiest microbial strains increasing when participants ate more whole grains. This study also found that higher rates of consumption of refined grain and gluten led to reduced microbial diversity.[161]

Overall, grains provide important nutrients that keep your cells functioning properly and support your overall health. So what is all the fuss about?

The Other Side of Grain

Let's address the three biggest problems with grains in our food supply and societies today: gluten, ultra-processing, and glyphosate (Roundup):

1. **The Gluten Problem:** Gluten is a complex of proteins in wheat, barley, and rye. This complex has become a subject of controversy due to how it can impact health. For some, particularly those with celiac disease, gluten triggers a severe immune response that damages the small intestine, leading to symptoms from digestive issues to fatigue. Even those without celiac disease can experience gluten sensitivity, where consuming gluten causes bloating, brain fog, and other discomforts. Gluten may also contribute to "leaky gut," a condition where the gut lining becomes porous, allowing toxins to enter the bloodstream and cause inflammation.

   Modern wheat has been hybridized to increase yield and improve baking qualities. These changes have resulted in grains with higher levels of gluten, which helps a loaf of bread stay together and gives it its springy, airy texture. Additionally, food manufacturers frequently add extra gluten to processed foods for texture and increased shelf life. This increased gluten exposure may be fueling the rise in gluten-related disorders. While many people can consume gluten without issue, the rising prevalence of gluten intolerance, celiac disease, and non-celiac gluten sensitivity suggests that our modern diets and the way we process wheat may be playing a role in exacerbating these conditions.[162]

2. **The Processing Problem:** Grains like wheat are often used in ultra-processed foods, undergoing changes that impact their nutritional value and effect on our bodies. Milling breaks down the grain's structure, leading to rapid glucose absorption and spikes in blood sugar and insulin, which can strain metabolic health and increase risks for conditions like insulin resistance and type 2 diabetes. Ultra-processing further strips the grain of its outer shell and germ, turning it from a complex carbohydrate into a simple one that digests quickly, prompting overeating due to a lack of fiber and nutrients. This can lead to increased body fat, raising the risk for cardiovascular diseases and certain cancers.[163,164]

3. **The Roundup (Glyphosate) Problem:** Glyphosate, a widely used herbicide and desiccant, is commonly applied to nonorganic grain crops before harvest to accelerate ripening and make harvest easier. However, this process leaves glyphosate residues in many commercial grain products, and the processed products made from them, raising significant health concerns. Research has linked glyphosate exposure to various health issues, including an increased risk of cancer, DNA mutations, and birth defects.[165]

    The International Agency for Research on Cancer, a part of the World Health Organization, has classified glyphosate as "probably carcinogenic to humans." Additionally, glyphosate is known to disrupt the gut microbiome, which plays a crucial role in human health by aiding digestion, supporting the immune system, and regulating various bodily functions. In addition to its effects on human health, glyphosate also affects soil microbiomes, leading to a decline in soil fertility and ecosystem health.[166]

How to Benefit from Grains

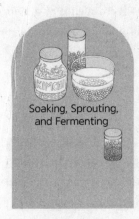

Soaking, Sprouting, and Fermenting

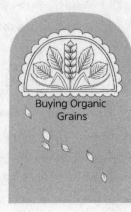

Buying Organic Grains

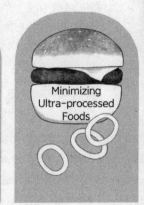

Minimizing Ultra-processed Foods

To help mitigate the effects of gluten sensitivity, exposure to glyphosate, and the impact of ultra-processed grains, there are several practical strategies you can adopt:

+ **Soaking, Sprouting, and Fermenting Grains:** Traditional practices like soaking, sprouting, and fermenting grains can enhance the grains' nutritional value and make them more digestible. For instance, fermenting grains into sourdough bread reduces the gluten content, which may help individuals with gluten sensitivity tolerate these foods better.[167]

+ **Buying Organic Grains:** Choosing organic grains and products made from them is another important strategy. Since organic farming standards prohibit the use of synthetic herbicides like glyphosate, consuming organic foods reduces your exposure to harmful chemicals.[168]

+ **Minimizing Consumption of Ultra-Processed Grain Products:** Limiting the intake of highly processed grain products such as white bread, sugary cereals, and pastries is crucial. These foods are often stripped of their natural nutrients and loaded with added sugars and unhealthy fats. A diet high in ultra-processed foods has been linked to various health issues, including obesity, type 2 diabetes, and cardiovascular diseases. Instead, opt for whole grains like brown rice, quinoa, and whole wheat products, which provide your body and your cells with more fiber, vitamins, and minerals.[169]

Are Legumes the Good Guys or the Bad Guys?

Recently, popular nutrition gurus have begun warning against eating legumes (beans, lentils, and peas) because they contain defensive proteins called lectins and nutrient storage molecules called phytates. Lectins and phytates can potentially cause inflammation, nutrient deficiencies, blood sugar spikes, poor bone health and tooth decay, digestive problems, and even allergic reactions. Diets such as paleo and keto have also encouraged strictly limiting legumes because they are relatively high in carbohydrates compared to other foods allowed on these diets.

I agree that the lectins, phytates, and even carbohydrates in legumes (and grains and some vegetables) can be harmful for health if they aren't handled correctly. But legumes, grains, and vegetables are well worth the "risk"—they are literal treasure troves of nutrients for you and your cells, and there are centuries-old methods for mitigating their negative effects. Let's learn what legumes can provide and how to handle them correctly:[170]

✦ Legumes, including beans, lentils, and chickpeas, are renowned for their high protein content, making them an excellent plant-based protein source. Protein allows for cell growth, repair, and maintenance, and the amino acids that make up these proteins are building blocks for muscle tissue, enzymes, and hormones, supporting overall health. For those following vegetarian or vegan diets, legumes are particularly valuable, as they provide a substantial amount of protein that is often lacking in non-animal-based diets. Including a variety of legumes in your diet ensures that you obtain a complete range of the amino acids necessary for optimal health.[171]

+ Legumes are also an excellent source of complex carbohydrates, which provide a steady and sustained release of energy throughout the day. Unlike simple carbohydrates, which can cause rapid spikes and crashes in blood sugar levels, the complex carbohydrates in legumes are digested slowly, helping to stabilize blood sugar levels and provide lasting energy. Additionally, the slow digestion of complex carbohydrates in legumes helps in managing weight by keeping you feeling full for longer periods.[172]

+ Legumes are full of nutrients! High in dietary fiber, a crucial component for digestive health, they promote regular bowel movements and prevent constipation. The fiber also regulates blood sugar levels and acts as a prebiotic, feeding the beneficial bacteria in your gut.[173]

+ Legumes are packed with essential nutrients such as folate, potassium, magnesium, and iron, which play vital roles in various bodily functions. Folate is crucial for DNA synthesis and cell division, making it especially important during periods of rapid growth, such as pregnancy and infancy. Potassium helps regulate fluid balance, muscle contractions, and nerve signals, while magnesium is involved in over three hundred chemical reactions, including energy production and protein synthesis. Iron is essential to the production of hemoglobin, the protein in red blood cells that transports oxygen throughout the body.[174]

+ Some legumes, such as black beans and kidney beans, are also rich in antioxidants, which help protect your cells from oxidative stress and damaging free radicals.[175]

How to Get the Benefits and Avoid the Concerns About Legumes

How to Benefit from Legumes

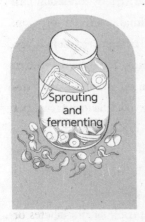
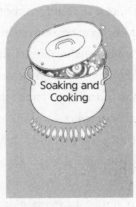
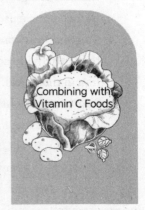

Sprouting and fermenting

Soaking and Cooking

Combining with Vitamin C Foods

✦ **Soaking and Cooking:** Soaking dried legumes such as beans, lentils, and chickpeas in water for several hours or overnight is a traditional method for breaking down antinutrients like lectins and phytates. By soaking and then thoroughly cooking the legumes through boiling, steaming, or pressure cooking, you not only reduce levels of antinutrients but also enhance the bioavailability of nutrients, making the legumes more digestible and nutritionally beneficial.[176] See Legume Soaking and Cooking Instructions in appendix 1 (page 305).

✦ **Sprouting and Fermenting:** These are powerful techniques that further reduce the levels of phytates and improve the digestibility of legumes. Sprouting involves soaking legumes until they begin to germinate or sprout, which increases their nutritional value and makes them easier to digest. Fermentation, a technique used to prepare foods like tempeh and miso, involves the breakdown of complex compounds in legumes by beneficial bacteria. This not only enhances their digestibility but also adds beneficial probiotics, which support gut health. These methods have been used for centuries in cultures around the world to improve the nutritional profile and digestibility of legumes.[177]

✦ **Combining with Foods that Contain Vitamin C:** Consuming legumes alongside foods high in vitamin C, such as tomatoes, bell peppers, or citrus fruits, can significantly enhance iron absorption. This simple dietary combination can help prevent iron deficiency, particularly in individuals who rely on plant-based foods for the iron in their diets. (For tasty recipes that combine legumes and vitamin C, check out Six-Can Chili (page 298) and Savory Crockpot Lentil Stew (page 315) in appendix 1.)[178]

What About Fruit?

Fruit contains sugar, which can be a problem for people with diabetes or insulin resistance and is avoided completely by low carbohydrate diets. For the rest of us, fruits and the nutrients they contain are powerhouses for your cells. Similar to those in grains, unprocessed, complex sugars like the ones found in fruit are very different than the ultra-processed white powder that you buy in bags at the grocery store.

Here are a few things to keep in mind as you consider the role of fruit in your diet:

✦ Fruits are a rich source of essential vitamins and minerals that play crucial roles in cellular metabolism, energy production, and overall cellular function. Vitamins such as vitamin C, vitamin A, and various B vitamins contribute to the proper functioning of metabolic pathways, support the immune system, and are vital for maintaining healthy skin, vision, and neurological function. Minerals like potassium, magnesium, and folate found in fruits are necessary for muscle function, nerve signaling, and DNA synthesis.[179]

✦ Many fruits are packed with antioxidants such as flavonoids, polyphenols, and vitamin C, which play a critical role in protecting your cells from oxidative stress. Oxidative stress, as we have learned, occurs when there is an imbalance between free radicals and antioxidants in the body, leading to cell damage and contributing to chronic diseases. The antioxidants in fruits help neutralize free radicals, reducing oxidative stress and inflammation. Additionally, some compounds in fruits have been found to have anticancer properties and immune-boosting functions.[180]

✦ Fruits are naturally high in water content, making them an excellent source of hydration. Regular consumption of fruits contributes to adequate hydration, which is vital for metabolic processes, joint lubrication, and maintaining healthy skin.[181]

✦ Fruits provide natural carbohydrates, which we have learned serve as a primary energy source for your cells. Unlike refined sugars found in processed foods, the sugars in fruits are accompanied by fiber, vitamins, and minerals, making them a healthier option for sustaining cellular energy. The fiber in fruits slows down the absorption of sugars, preventing rapid spikes and crashes in blood sugar levels, making fruits ideal if you're looking for a natural and nutritious energy boost.[182]

How to Benefit from Fruit

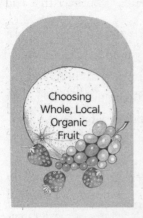
Choosing Whole, Local, Organic Fruit

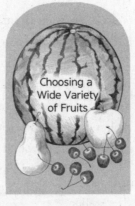
Choosing a Wide Variety of Fruits

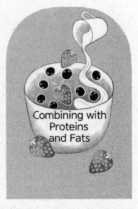
Combining with Proteins and Fats

✦ **Opt for Whole Fruits:** Whole fruits contain more fiber and fewer added sugars than fruit juices or processed fruit snacks.

✦ **Shop Organic (and Local):** If you are able to access it, organic fruit will reduce your exposure to harmful pesticides and synthetic chemicals. In addition, locally grown fruit—especially seasonal fruit—is at its nutritional peak and will often be fresher and taste better than fruit that has traveled long distances to reach your kitchen. (Whether or not your fruit is organic, make sure to wash it thoroughly under running water, especially if eating it with the skin on.)

✦ **Enjoy a Diverse Range of Fruits:** This ensures you will benefit from a wider variety of vitamins, minerals, and antioxidants. Choose fruits with edible skins or seeds, such as apples, berries, and pears, to increase your fiber intake, which supports digestive health and helps regulate blood sugar levels.

✦ **Combine Fruits with Proteins and Fats:** Foods rich in protein and fat include Greek yogurt, nuts, or seeds, as well as avocado and nut butter. These foods can help balance blood sugar levels and help you feel full. Blend fruits into smoothies with leafy greens, protein, and healthy fats for a nutritious meal or snack.[183]

What Role Should Vegetables Play in the Diet?

Recently I watched a video posted by a social media influencer that had garnered millions of views. In a conspiratorial tone, he warned followers that eating vegetables could kill them. Surprised? Me, too. Where did this kind of information come from?

Vegetables are being debated due to conflicting views on many hot topics like the safety of lectins and the reduced benefits of raw versus cooked vegetables (and vice versa). All these concerns are valid, but there are ways to manage the concerns while still reaping the benefits vegetables provide.

The well-established health benefits of consuming plant-based foods, including grains, legumes, fruits, and vegetables, are supported by a substantial body of scientific evidence. This evidence shows a reduced risk of cardiovascular diseases, including heart attack and stroke, improved digestion, better blood sugar regulation, and healthy cholesterol levels for those that eat plants.[184]

Plants are also linked to lower incidences of certain cancers, such as colorectal and breast cancer, due to the high levels of antioxidants and phytochemicals that they contain, which help protect cells from damage and reduce inflammation. Moreover, consuming a variety of plant foods can help maintain a healthy weight, as these foods are typically lower in calories and higher in nutrients, helping you to feel full and turn off your appestat after you've eaten. The benefits also extend to improved gut health, as the fiber in plant-based foods feeds beneficial gut bacteria, supporting a healthy microbiome that plays a crucial role in overall health, including immune function and mental well-being.

So, what is there to argue about? A lot, apparently! Two of the most contentious topics center on lectins and on the effect of cooking on vegetables' nutritional content.

+ **The Lectin Debate:** The debate surrounding lectins in vegetables centers on their potential health risks versus their role in a healthy diet. Lectins are a type of protein "antinutrient" found in many plant-based foods, including the legumes and grains we have already discussed as well certain other foods like tomatoes and potatoes. Lectins can bind to carbohydrates in the digestive tract, potentially interfering with nutrient absorption and leading to digestive issues such as bloating, gas, and even more severe conditions like "leaky gut." Some suggest that lectins, particularly when consumed in large amounts or in their raw form, may contribute to autoimmune disorders and inflammation.

On the other hand, many nutrition experts emphasize that the concerns about lectins are largely overblown when it comes to the average diet. They point out that the vast majority of lectins are deactivated through proper cooking methods, such as boiling, soaking, or fermenting, which significantly reduce any potential negative effects. Moreover, vegetables and legumes, which are high in lectins, are also rich in essential nutrients, fiber, and antioxidants that provide significant health benefits, including reducing the risk of chronic diseases like heart disease, diabetes, and cancer. The consensus in the scientific community is that the health benefits of consuming these foods far outweigh the potential risks associated with lectins, especially when the foods are prepared properly.[185, 186]

✦ **Raw Versus Cooked Vegetables:** The debate over raw versus cooked vegetables revolves around the nutritional differences and health benefits of consuming vegetables in their raw state compared to their cooked form. Proponents of raw vegetables argue that cooking can destroy certain heat-sensitive nutrients, such as vitamin C and some B vitamins, as well as enzymes that may aid in digestion and enhance nutrient absorption. They suggest that eating vegetables raw ensures that these nutrients remain intact, providing maximum health benefits. On the other hand, advocates for cooking vegetables highlight that cooking can break down the tough cell walls of plants, making certain nutrients, like lycopene in tomatoes and beta-carotene in carrots, more bioavailable. Additionally, cooking can reduce or eliminate certain antinutrients, like lectins and oxalates, which can interfere with nutrient absorption and cause digestive issues. The general consensus is that a balanced diet should include a variety of both raw and cooked vegetables to maximize nutrient intake and health benefits.[187]

How to Benefit from Vegetables

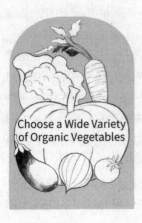
Choose a Wide Variety of Organic Vegetables

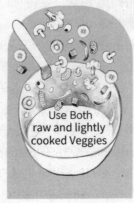
Use Both raw and lightly cooked Veggies

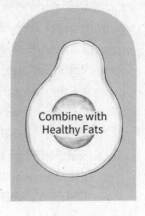
Combine with Healthy Fats

✦ **Include a Diverse Range of Vegetables in Your Diet:** This includes leafy greens, cruciferous vegetables (like broccoli and cauliflower), root vegetables (such as carrots and sweet potatoes), and colorful bell peppers. Each type offers unique vitamins, minerals, and antioxidants.[188]

✦ **Choose Organic and Local:** When feasible, favor organic vegetables to reduce your exposure to pesticides and synthetic chemicals. Additionally, selecting locally grown produce ensures freshness and supports sustainable agriculture practices.

✦ **Eat Raw and Lightly Cooked Vegetables:** Opt for gentle methods of cooking like steaming, sautéing, or roasting with minimal added fats to preserve vegetables' nutritional value and deactivate lectins. Fermented vegetables such as sauerkraut, kimchi, and pickles are also beneficial for wellness, as they are rich in probiotics and enzymes that support gut health and digestion.

✦ **Incorporate Healthy Fats:** Fats like olive oil, avocado, or nuts ensure that certain nutrients in vegetables are absorbed by your body.

How to Choose Healthy Food

It can be extremely difficult to know when the nutritional choices you are making are truly contributing to your wellness—or not. One major problem exacerbating unhealthy "wellness" choices is misleading labels and health claims perpetuated by food and beverage companies. These can confuse consumers and obscure the true nutritional value of foods. The food industry spends billions of dollars each year on marketing and advertising campaigns designed to promote certain products as healthy or "natural" choices. Terms like "organic," "gluten-free," and "all-natural" are often used to imply healthfulness, even though they may not always be indicative of a food's overall nutritional quality. With so much information, it can be hard for the average person, who isn't a doctor or nutritionist, to determine what makes a food nutritious and good for their cells and body.

The field of nutrition is constantly evolving, but the influx of information can sometimes lead to contradictory recommendations. Media sensationalism and cherry-picking of scientific studies can further contribute to the confusion, as headlines proclaiming the latest "superfood" or "diet miracle" can overshadow less exciting discussions about simple, balanced nutrition. Some recent headlines found online at this writing:

- ✦ "Could a Low-Cal Keto Diet Help Ease Acne?"
- ✦ "Could Having 'Skinny' Fat Cells Encourage Weight Gain?"
- ✦ "More Data Suggests 'Ultraprocessed' Foods Can Shorten Your Life"

To move beyond confusion, and to be able to embrace plants as the mainstay of wellness, here are some important definitions:

Organic: Foods labeled as "organic" must adhere to USDA standards, which prohibit the use of synthetic fertilizers, sewage sludge as fertilizer, irradiation, and genetic engineering.

What you need to know: Organic food is often marketed as healthier, and in many cases, it is. However, the term "organic" itself does not mean higher nutritional value. Organic farming can still use natural fertilizers, pesticides, and herbicides. This offers some challenges because there is variability in what is considered a "natural" product, and some might still pose risks to health or the environment. For example, "natural" copper-based fungicides can accumulate in the soil and become toxic over time.

Natural/All-natural: This label indicates that the product is free from artificial ingredients, colors, or flavors.

What you need to know: There are no regulations on the use of the term "natural," meaning that it can legally be applied to almost any food. It's frequently used for marketing purposes.

Non-GMO/GMO-free: Products with this label do not contain genetically modified organisms (GMOs). Genetic modifications are typically conducted to increase organisms' resistance to pests and weeds.

What you need to know: Some products might be labeled non-GMO as a marketing tactic even when there isn't a GMO version, such as GMO-free water. Are GMO containing foods safe and beneficial to consume? The jury is still out. There are thousands of research articles related to genetically modified organisms (GMOs) in food, including both supportive and critical perspectives on their safety, nutritional content, and environmental impact.

The Eating Well Filter

The Environmental Working Group (EWG) is a nonprofit organization focused on environmental research and advocacy in the United States. They assess the safety of chemicals in consumer products, evaluate pesticide levels in produce, advocate for sustainable agriculture, and more. Each year they publish their "Dirty Dozen" and "Clean Fifteen" reports, which rank fruits and vegetables based on their pesticide residue levels. (Go to ewg.org for the latest list.)

Dirty Dozen: The dirty dozen identifies the twelve fruits and vegetables with the highest pesticide residues in the food chain for that year in the US. These are items that EWG suggests buying organic whenever possible to reduce exposure to potentially harmful chemicals. Examples include strawberries, spinach, kale, apples, grapes, and tomatoes.

Clean Fifteen: In contrast, the Clean Fifteen highlights the fifteen fruits and vegetables with the lowest pesticide residues. These are items that EWG suggests are safest to consume conventionally grown if buying organic is not feasible. Examples include avocados, sweet corn, pineapple, onions, and cauliflower.

These lists help you and I make informed choices about which produce items we should purchase organic to minimize pesticide exposure, and which we can save some money on and confidently purchase conventionally grown. For me, this takes the worry out of choosing safe plants for my family. If possible, I select organic versions of the Dirty Dozen and don't worry as much about things on the Clean Fifteen list. This is one component of something I call the Eating Well Filter. This filtering process helps you navigate through the confusion to find the foods your body and cells need. This is a "good, better, best" filter that can help guide your food choices.

Is every food that makes it through this filter the absolute best, cleanest, purest food you can consume? Not by any stretch of the imagination. And that's okay! Your body is amazing at helping you, and it can mitigate some of the consequences of eating non-optimal foods. After all, keeping you alive and functioning at your best is your body's only job! It works at it 24/7, with systems that support your wellness despite the hazardous world you live in. This doesn't mean your body will just "deal" with a nonstop diet of diet soda, processed meals and French fries; there's a limit to what your body can protect you from and adapt to. But you do need to recognize your body's innate ability to help you be well. As Sarah's example illustrates, sometimes stressing too much about "perfect" nutrition can reduce wellness, too.

The Eating Well filter provides a simple and practical way to make healthier dietary decisions by putting foods into three ranked categories. Here's how it works:

Good: This represents the baseline or minimum acceptable choice. Compared to many alternatives, it's typically a healthier option for your cells, but it may still have some drawbacks. For example:

+ Choosing whole grains over refined grains
+ Selecting low-fat or reduced-sugar versions of processed foods
+ Including a variety of fruits and vegetables in your meals
+ Choosing organic for Dirty Dozen foods when possible

Better: This represents an improved choice that offers greater nutritional benefits or fewer drawbacks for your cells compared to the "good" option. It typically involves selecting foods that are less processed, higher in nutrients, and more aligned with your health goals. For example:

+ Choosing whole, unprocessed foods over heavily processed foods
+ Selecting organic produce for the Dirty Dozen as well as other foods that you eat the surface of, like apples, tomatoes, lettuce, and spinach
+ Making a conscious choice to eat foods with minimal added sugars, salt, and unhealthy fats

Best: This represents the optimal choice that provides the highest nutritional value and medicinal benefits for your cells along with the fewest potential drawbacks. It often involves selecting foods that are minimally processed, rich in nutrients and plant medicines, and supportive of overall health and well-being. For example:

+ Choosing fresh, whole foods like fruits, vegetables, whole grains, nuts, seeds, legumes, and other plants that have added health benefits, such as garlic
+ Choosing organic foods as often as possible
+ Opting for foods with little to no added sugars, unhealthy fats, artificial additives, and preservatives

By now, you should be well on your way to understanding the importance of plants to wellness. But what do you do if you can't wander the hills picking blueberries in the spring or your finances don't allow for exclusively organic produce? Can you get these benefits from your blueberry-free apartment in New York City or from a bottle of whole food–based supplements? The Eating Well Filter can help you answer these questions. (Hint: the answer is yes.) While not as potent, a combination of supplements and packaged and fresh foods can go a long way when the optimal nutritional options are not available. Remember, "good" foods are still good. Don't beat yourself up because you can't get the "best" foods all the time. You may have financial, access, or other constraints that aren't in your control. If you do, don't worry. Your body and cells will do their part. This isn't a "lesser" way to eat well and is largely how I have structured how my family eats and gets nutrients.

Eating Well in Real Life

Now let's take some of these concepts and apply them to real life. As I've shared, I have struggled with gut health over the years. I think it partly has to do with exposure I've had in the dental office to mercury and other chemical toxins, but I think it can also be attributed to stress, to genetics and just to life! As I visited different practitioners, read books and blogs, and looked online for answers, I became very overwhelmed. One well-meaning practitioner even told me to remove not only gluten, but also corn, eggs, dairy, meat, vinegar, and pickles from my diet. I went home, thought about this diet, and cried. I felt bad for myself. I didn't know what I was going to eat—even though I am educated and experienced in diet, cooking, and dietary alternatives. I looked at the recommended "don't eat" list and thought, "If I can't do this, very few people can."

The next time I went back to this practitioner's office, I stopped to chat with her receptionist. I asked if people were actually successful on this diet. She honestly answered, "All I do, all day long, is field questions from people who say, 'I can't do this! How do I do this? What do I eat? There's nothing left.'" After this conversation, I knew I wasn't alone! This huge jump into new foods and a new way of eating was like going from kindergarten to graduate school in one day, and it's just not possible, no matter how well meaning and dedicated you are. That's why you can take the Eating Well Filter's guidelines and work through them slowly, as life allows, giving yourself grace and room to change as you go.

Here are some examples of using the Eating Well Filter while choosing your food:

	Good	Better	Best
Oats	Granola bar	Flavored oatmeal	Steel cut oats
Yogurt	Sweetened yogurt drink	Flavored yogurt	Plain yogurt
Green beans	Canned green beans	Frozen green beans	Fresh organic green beans
Peaches	Canned peaches in water	Dried peaches	Fresh organic peaches
Greens	Iceberg lettuce	Romaine lettuce	Organic spinach
Almonds	Snacking almonds with seasonings	Almond butter	Sprouted almonds

For more ideas and guidance on applying the Eating Well Filter, go to www.livingwellwithdrmichelle.com/book.

These are the exact recommendations I gave my patient Polly as she started working toward eating well for better cell and overall health. She was completely overwhelmed. She had started purchasing packaged foods and frozen foods to save time, because even a little change like buying vegetables and cutting them up to put in a meal felt like too much. She wasn't even sure how to use a chef's knife correctly or which vegetables to buy. She watched a bunch of shows on the Cooking Channel, but realized very quickly they weren't about real, "in-your-own-kitchen-every-day"–type cooking.

When Polly started working with the Eating Well Filter and plan, she asked if there was a way to use some packaged goods but turn them into homemade dishes. As you can see from the chart above, the answer is *yes*! The "homemade-only" way is not possible in many of our lives. This concept is what I call "homemade-ish": using the right prepackaged goods, primarily plants with some scratch ingredients, to make meals that help your cells and body stay well, while staying within your time, budget, and skill constraints.

Eating Well with Prepackaged Foods

These packaged foods can speed up the making of healthy meals, while retaining most of their nutritional value.

+ Canned beans, including green beans
+ Canned tomatoes
+ Canned broths
+ Frozen veggies and mixes (without sauce)
+ Packaged pastas
+ Rice and other grains
+ Premade tortillas
+ Packaged corn chips
+ Packaged granola bars
+ Some granolas
+ Packaged noodles

+ Condiments
+ Salsa
+ Pickles
+ Frozen fruit

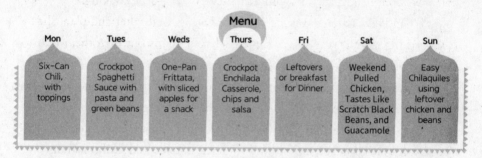

Mon	Tues	Weds	**Menu** Thurs	Fri	Sat	Sun
Six-Can Chili, with toppings	Crockpot Spaghetti Sauce with pasta and green beans	One-Pan Frittata, with sliced apples for a snack	Crockpot Enchilada Casserole, chips and salsa	Leftovers or breakfast for Dinner	Weekend Pulled Chicken, Tastes Like Scratch Black Beans, and Guacamole	Easy Chilaquiles using leftover chicken and beans

A sample meal plan developed using the Eating Well Filter.

All recipes in this meal plan can be found in appendix 1 of this book and online at www.resources.livingwellbook.com.

By using the "good, better, best" Eating Well Filter, you can gradually improve your dietary habits and make choices, including eating more plants, that support your cells' health and your wellness over the long term. Simply stated, plants provide the building blocks your body needs to stay healthy and return to health when needed.

Chapter 6
Keyhole Concepts

+ Plants give your cells nutrients that they need, like antioxidants, minerals, fiber, and other compounds.
+ To truly harness the power of plants, we need to use them in their whole, unprocessed form: food that is as close to its natural state as possible. Your cells work best when using whole foods as fuel.

+ Nutrients found in whole foods interact in complex ways within the body, creating synergistic effects that cannot be replicated if those nutrients are isolated and used individually in processed foods or supplements.
+ The Eating Well Filter helps you easily make choices about what to eat to nourish your cells without getting overstressed.

CHAPTER 7

Earth

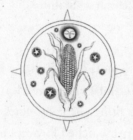

In our twenty-first-century world, many people are increasingly losing their connection with the earth. Instead of spending time outside, working or playing in nature, they spend time in their offices. Many urban landscapes are full of pavement, with very few trees. People think they have their "feet on the ground," but comfortable, insulating shoes with thick rubber soles actually separate them from contact with the earth. This physical contact with the earth provides your cells and body with electrons that help power up energy generation and tamp down inflammation. The earth also provides minerals called electrolytes that carry signals between cells. You can get these electrolytes from plants that have been grown in healthy soil. Nutrients, energy, and sustenance come from the earth, and you will learn how to partner with the earth for better cellular wellness.

Lost Connection with the Earth

Chief Arvol Looking Horse, a respected spiritual leader of the Lakota people, remembers and teaches of a time when people and the land were connected. Indigenous peoples understand that the soil is not merely a medium for growing crops; it is the source of life and sustenance. In many indigenous cultures, including the Lakota, ceremonies and rituals are performed to honor the earth and maintain harmony with the natural world. Reconnecting with the land and understanding the kinship that all humans have with it is essential to maintaining the wellness of your cells and body. The earth is the source of all the electrons every cell requires to continue functioning.

When I started on my journey to heal my body and cells, I learned that I needed more of the cellular energy you learned about in chapter 5. I also learned that electrons bring energy, wellness, and improved function to every cellular system. As I searched for ways to improve my wellness, a friend told me about a concept called "grounding" or "Earthing." Grounding isn't a new practice or concept. Grounding something electrically means connecting it to the earth using a conductor, a material that electricity can flow through easily. Like a lightning rod on a building, this conductor gives electricity a safe path to the ground, preventing electrical surges or faults from causing damage to equipment or injury to people.

Electrical Grounding

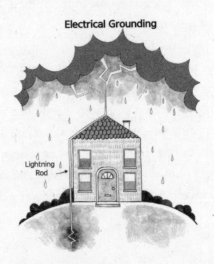

Lightning Rod

Grounding a Person

The concept of grounding a person recently gained popularity due to the efforts of a man named Clint Ober. Ober had previously worked in the cable television industry, and so he understood the need to "ground" cable signals for static-free TV reception. During his retirement, Ober had chronic back pain, and he began to wonder if humans would benefit from grounding, too. He remembered visiting a Native American friend growing up whose mother advised them to remove their shoes, warning, "They'll make you sick." Now that he was unwell, her advice jumped out to him, and he realized that modern footwear with rubber or synthetic soles was keeping him from touching the earth, even when walking on it.

Using a makeshift system of duct tape, wires, and a grounding rod, Ober connected his bed to the ground. The first night he slept in this "grounded" bed, he woke at dawn, shocked to find that he had slept through the night without waking and that his pain was nearly gone. Something had helped his cells during the night, turning off his body's cellular signal for pain. Encouraged by his experience, Ober began to share and test his grounding process with friends, who reported similar cell health and symptom improvements.[189] Motivated by these positive outcomes, Ober organized a formal study to research what he called Earthing, and other studies have followed. These studies have found that grounding appears to improve sleep, reduce pain, reduce stress, quiet the fight-or-flight response in the body, improve the heart's ability to respond to stressors, speed wound healing, and even thin the blood, reducing the chance of clotting and strokes.[190]

While Clint Ober is recognized for popularizing Earthing, he acknowledges that the practice of connecting to the ground isn't his invention, but rather has a long history in Native American spirituality. Luther Standing Bear, another Lakota leader, described the profound relationship his people have with the soil: "The old people came literally to love the soil and they sat or reclined on the ground with a feeling of being close to a mothering power. It was good for the skin to touch the earth . . . The soil was soothing, strengthening, cleansing, and healing."[191]

The Science of Earthing

Modern scientific research is only now catching up with these traditional practices. The science behind Earthing is rooted in the idea that the earth's surface has an abundant supply of electrons and has a natural negative electric charge.[192] Positive and negative charges are constantly traveling between different parts of the human body. The positive charges are called free radicals, and they are both produced by your internal cellular mitochondria and build up internally because of pollutants and electronic radiation from household appliances, mobile phones, Wi-Fi, microwaves, and cell towers.[193] As you may remember, these free radicals are highly reactive molecules that strip electrons from healthy tissue, resulting in damage, in a process called oxidative stress.

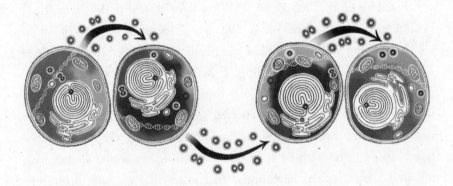

Free radicals steal electrons from different structures in the cell, including the cell membranes, making them less stable and more prone to rupture, which can lead to cell death. This accelerates the aging process, both internally and externally, and can manifest as wrinkles, reduced organ function, and an increased susceptibility to age-related diseases. Oxidative stress can also trigger an inflammatory response in the body, which can damage proteins, causing them to become misshapen or dysfunctional. Most concerningly, these free radicals damage your DNA, leading to mutations and epigenetic changes that can increase the risk for cellular diseases, including cardiovascular disease, cancer, and neurodegenerative disorders like Alzheimer's and Parkinson's disease.

To neutralize these free radicals, your body needs antioxidants from fruits and vegetables as well as a constant supply of negatively charged particles called electrons.[194] This influx of electrons stops the oxidation reactions that cause damage to your cells—like the air turning an apple brown after it's cut. Restoring and maintaining the body's internal electrical environment, this flow of electrons stabilizes cell systems at the deepest levels, reducing inflammation, pain, and stress, and improving blood flow, immune function, energy, and sleep.

The good news is that there is a limitless, free source of those electrons banked and ready for you to withdraw.[195] That electron bank is the earth. When you make direct contact with the earth, those free electrons flow along the skin and into the cells in the body, counteracting free radicals. The abundant negative electrical charge that your body gains also pushes environmental electricity, like the electrical fields from devices like cell phones and Wi-Fi, away from the body. These fields interfere with cells, increase stress on the body, and affect sleep and hormones, potentially leading to health issues over time.

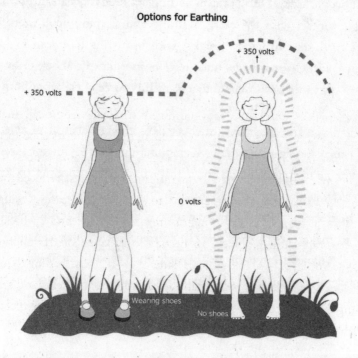

Options for Earthing

+ 350 volts

+ 350 volts

0 volts

Wearing shoes

No shoes

Numerous recent studies show that this direct contact with the earth, whether outdoors barefoot or indoors connected to grounded systems, can be a simple and effective way to combat inflammation. Chronic inflammatory diseases have been recognized as "the most significant cause of death in the world today," with more than 50 percent of all deaths being attributable to inflammation-related diseases, including heart disease, stroke, cancer, diabetes, chronic kidney disease, liver disease, and autoimmune and neurological conditions.[196] It's a good thing, then, that the earth we live on is the original painkiller and anti-inflammatory! Simply putting your skin into contact with the earth is an easy, natural way to support biochemical and physiological processes that promote cell wellness.[197]

Modern Age Electron Deficiency

Because most people in our modern world are disconnected from the earth, we are missing out on these free wellness benefits found right under our feet. The term "electron-deficient" might perfectly describe the condition of most people today. During the preceding hundreds of years, people lived in direct contact with the earth, walking and sleeping on it every day. Today's earth-disconnected lifestyles, with insulating footwear, high-rise buildings, and elevated beds, must have been a bit of a shock to human cells and systems that were used to a plentiful source of electrons both day and night.

When you feel like you just don't have enough energy, or can't get enough energy, it's possible that you are suffering from having too few electrons flowing to your cells and body. Think back to the "hot potato" transfer of electrons that the cells use to create ATP, or energy, that we learned about in chapter 5. Having more electrons available increases your cells' ability to make energy, improves the efficiency of cellular signaling, and helps cells recover from damage.[198] People often report that after they start grounding or Earthing, they feel and look healthier and younger, have less pain, and even have a more positive mood. Electrons from the earth are the best antioxidants, with no side effects because our bodies evolved to use this version of the earth's nutrition.[199] The best part is that this "electric nutrition" is free, easy to use, and achieves rapid results.[200]

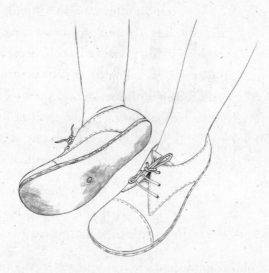

Earthing shoes, with leather soles and a copper plug, can help release positive ions back into the earth. This can help with stress, promote better sleep, reduce inflammation, promote healing, reduce pain, and increase blood flow.

These electrons are a non-pharmaceutical therapy that has been dubbed "vitamin G" (for grounding).[201] How can you access these electrons? The simplest way to get more vitamin G is to walk barefoot outdoors; a grassy park, yard, or sandy beach are ideal locations.[202] In other areas, you can wear electron-conductive Earthing shoes to protect your feet while simultaneously gaining electrons through the soles.

The most convenient and popular way to connect with the ground is from inside your home or office while you are working, relaxing, or sleeping. Grounding or Earthing products have an imbedded cord that can be plugged into the ground port on a wall outlet (the round hole beneath the part you plug a two-prong electrical cord into) or attached to a grounding rod placed in the soil outside. Grounding sheets, mats, pads, body bands, and patches are all available to be used while sitting or sleeping.

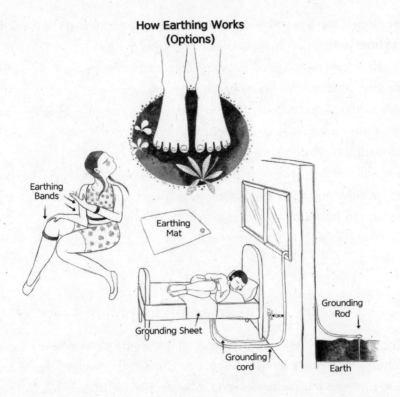

How Earthing Works (Options)

Earthing Bands

Earthing Mat

Grounding Sheet

Grounding cord

Grounding Rod

Earth

I witnessed just how powerful these products can be after my friend experienced a particularly difficult knee surgery. The surgical sites didn't heal well, and started to swell, redden, and weep fluid. My friend was put on three rounds of ever stronger antibiotics without relief. Her knee was too sore to stand or walk on, so she spent her days sitting in a recliner, often with tears streaming down her face from the pain. I suggested she try putting grounding bands around her leg to bring healing electrons to the site. She was willing to try anything, so I brought her two grounding bands and wrapped one around her leg above the knee and another below. I attached the bands to cords that plugged into the grounding port of a nearby wall outlet. Afterwards, I stayed to chat for a few minutes, and I was surprised when she nodded off to sleep while we were talking. Free from pain for the first time in months, she slept for hours that afternoon, and then all through the night. She didn't experience immediate, 100 percent relief, but it was enough to help her get out of the chair. Within two weeks, the swelling had gone down, she was slowly moving around her home, and she was nearly free from pain.

How long do you need to be in contact with the earth for this to be effective? Studies show an immediate increase in electrical activity in the body as soon as contact begins, and medical infrared imaging shows that inflammation begins to subside within thirty minutes of connecting with the earth.[203] I would recommend either sleeping with an earthing sheet or pad, which will give you six to eight hours of "vitamin G" per night, or aiming for thirty minutes of contact four to seven times per week for reduction in pain and inflammation and improvement in immune function.[204]

How long do you need to continue the practice? As long as you want to be well!

The Earth Calms Inflammation

When people visit my dental practice and I see they are suffering from problems with inflammation, my first and simplest recommendation for them is to reconnect with the earth. One memorable patient, John, came to see me for treatment for snoring. Because we look in the mouth and at the head and neck, dentists are a great resource for treating and eliminating snoring. With advanced radiographic technology, we can assess the root cause of snoring, which is often connected to the size, shape, or condition of the mouth, and can provide treatment for snoring that corrects these root causes rather than bandaging the problem with a CPAP.[205]

John was looking for these kinds of answers. He was diabetic, had swollen legs and feet, and snored like a freight train at night. During my evaluation, I found a few correctable problems for John. His mouth had developed with too little room for his teeth and his tongue, leading to his tongue falling backward when he was sleeping at night. This blocked his airflow, which causes not only snoring but also increased inflammation and overall body distress.

John was excited to start wearing an appliance to help expand his mouth and make room for everything to fit. But in the meantime, I suggested that he sleep on grounding sheets to address his inflammation and swelling with a steady supply of the earth's electrons. John was skeptical but agreed to try, and after using them for one week, he and his wife were shocked to report his snoring was nearly gone. Those extra electrons energized his cells and body, leading to easier breathing, which improved his sleep quality.[206] After a couple of months of use, John reported another surprising side effect: Earthing had impacted his blood sugar levels.[207] He was routinely measuring lower levels when testing his blood during the day, which made it easier to control his diabetes. One simple, inexpensive solution had led to a cascade of health improvements throughout his body.

Some ways you can reconnect with the earth:
+ Take your socks off when you are outside.
+ Walk outside, even if it's just on soil or grass in your backyard.
+ If you need a chair when you sit, keep your feet on the ground when outside.
+ Swim in the ocean or walk on the beach.
+ Garden without gloves.
+ If you can't get to the earth, you can try grounding patches, sheets, mats, bands, shoes, and socks. They work by physically connecting you to the earth through the grounding port on your electrical outlets, a wire and a rod in the ground, or a disk on the sole of your shoe or sock.

Bringing Electrons to the Cells

Once free electrons enter your body, they need to be routed and carried to the right cells. The earth supplies the electrons, but how do those electrons get to the cells where they are needed? The answer is electrolytes. They carry electrons to the cells that need them and play a critical role in your body's cell signaling.

When my children were younger, I decided it would be good for our family to have some basic survival skills we could fall back on if needed. I hired a wilderness survival specialist to take my husband, myself, and our four children (ages seven to fourteen at the time) on a "survival weekend."

We packed up the few things he allowed each of us to bring—a sleeping bag, water bottle, metal cup for cooking and eating, and a pocketknife—and headed for some desolate brown hills in central Utah a few hours away. We were going to be learning how to survive off the land: how to make a fire without matches, purify water on that fire, gather natural materials for a shelter, and forage from stream banks and dusty hollows for food.

We started the weekend in good spirits. We were excited to learn how to make a "friction fire," mastered weaving rope out of plants, and found that the roots of a plant we called a cattail didn't taste too bad. While making her woven rope, my seven-year-old daughter, inexperienced at using a pocketknife, slipped and cut her finger. Using what we had, I bandaged her finger with a fuzzy leaf from a native mullein plant and held the leaf in place with a hair tie.

That night, exhausted, my daughter and I crawled into our homemade cedar-branch shelter. During the night, my daughter woke up and vomited. She hadn't eaten anything other than cattail roots and boiled water all day, so I assumed that those had upset her stomach. She vomited twice more during the night, and in the morning, I woke up feeling worried about her cut finger and her health. My husband hiked back to our car to retrieve some trail mix for her. She ate the mix, drank some more water, and threw up again. She was still pale, shaky, and weak. We had been planning to stay another night, but as the day went on, my daughter was becoming concerningly lethargic. We carried her as we walked along the hills looking for something to eat, and she begged to lie down and sleep.

At that point, we decided to cut our weekend short and take her home. Starving, dirty, and tired, we were all excited when the first sign of life—and food—came into view. Knowing we had very empty stomachs to fill, we excitedly pulled into an Asian buffet restaurant. My daughter has always loved the salty, savory taste of miso soup, and that was all she wanted at the restaurant. She quickly drank one bowl of soup, then another, and then a third. After the third bowl was empty, the color had come back to her cheeks, she was joining in the "war stories" my other kids were telling about the weekend and their mother's crazy ideas, and she was asking for more food.

Why did miso soup make her feel so much better so quickly? Electrolytes!

Signs of Low Electrolytes:

✦ Confusion and irritability

✦ Diarrhea or constipation

✦ Fatigue

✦ Headaches

✦ Irregular or fast heart rate (arrhythmia)

✦ Muscle cramps, muscle spasms, or weakness

✦ Nausea and vomiting

✦ Numbness or tingling in limbs, fingers, and toes

Sports participants, weekend warriors, and people who work outside all talk about "needing electrolytes" after sweating, playing, or working in the hot sun. Most of you know you can find these electrolytes in bottles of sweetly salty, colorful liquid at the grocery store or gas station, but do you know what electrolytes are or why your cells need them?

Chemically, electrolytes are substances that have a natural positive or negative electrical charge and conduct electricity when dissolved in water. The term "electrolyte" comes from "electro-" (related to electricity) and "-lyte" (from "lysis," meaning to break apart). When electrolytes dissolve, they break into positively and negatively charged particles called ions, which carry electrical charges all over the body.

How Electrolytes Help the Body

Electrolytes are the carriers for the electrons that are passed from cell to cell as your cells talk to or signal one another. An adult's body is about 60 percent water, and this high water content allows ions to flow in and out of cells easily. These electrolytes coordinate essential life functions, including:

+ Running the electrical workings of the brain, heart, and nervous system.
+ Helping your body regulate chemical reactions.
+ Governing everything from your heartbeat and immune responses to your nerve and muscle function.
+ Maintaining the balance between fluids inside and outside your cells.[208]

Like electrons, electrolytes are found in the earth, and your body gets them from what you eat and drink. Sodium, potassium, chloride, magnesium, calcium, phosphate, and bicarbonates are all electrolytes. These electrolytes turn cells into tiny batteries. The number of electrolytes inside and outside the cells creates an electrical charge, like positive and negative ends of a battery. When one of these molecules enters or exits the cell, it brings its electrons with it, and when electrons move, they create electricity, which helps conduct signals between cells throughout the body. Looking at the blue sky, moving your muscles as you walk down stairs, and your rhythmic heartbeat are all bodily functions that electrolyte movement makes happen. Some common electrolytes include:

+ Sodium (Na+) and potassium (K+), which travel back and forth across the cell membrane to fire nerves and to transport nutrients in and waste products out.
+ Calcium (Ca++) ions, which cause a muscle to contract, assist with the way DNA is read, moderate the secretion of hormones and other signaling molecules from cells, and even help with how a cell metabolizes nutrients.
+ Hydrogen (H+) ions, which drive the production of ATP we learned about in chapter 5, and whose movement—alongside bicarbonate (HCO3-) ions—helps regulate the cell's pH.
+ Sodium (Na+) and chloride (Cl-), which help maintain water balance in your body.

What Electrolytes Do for Cells

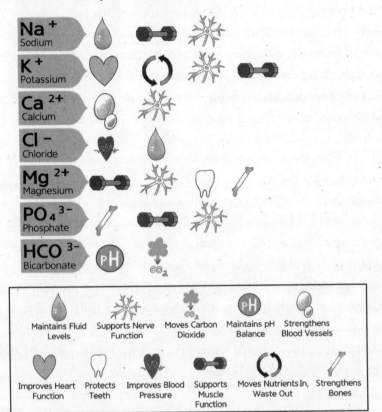

These are just a few of the hundreds of body functions
that happen because of electrolytes.[209]

Your body loses electrolytes through urine and sweat. If you've ever run your sweaty hand against parched, dry lips after working hard, you know sweat is salty. Urine and blood are, too. Sodium and chlorine dissolve in water, and so when water leaves your body, these ions leave with it, making sweat taste salty. This can lead to trouble when more water and electrolytes exit the body than are replaced, as my daughter experienced in the wilderness.

In the wilderness, my daughter's body began running out of electrolytes, and it struggled to maintain all the functions that are run by these ions. She had been eating very little and sweating a lot, and she had lost blood from her cut finger. We made sure she was drinking, so she avoided dehydration, but the water further diluted the electrolytes left in her system and led to her worrisome symptoms. Because our daughter was small and didn't have large stores of these electrolytes to call on, she felt the effect of these deficiencies before the rest of us. The vomiting, lethargy, and desire for sleep were all signs of electrolyte imbalance. As the salt left her body along with the water, her cells slowly lost their ability to signal each other properly.

We learned a lot about my daughter and about the importance of electrolytes on that ill-fated survival trip weekend. For a few years before this experience, she had been complaining of occasional sharp pains in her chest. Now those pains made sense. She is very sensitive to electrolyte imbalances in her cells, and those pains were her chest muscles letting her know their electrolyte levels were low. Nowadays we are always stocked up on electrolyte drink mixes, and she always has a few on hand when playing sports or pushing herself physically. While those drink mixes and grocery store sports drinks are a good source of these much-needed electrolytes and are very convenient, they aren't the best source of electrons. The best source is simply the earth.

Partnership with the Earth

Those of us living earth-disconncted lifestyles have almost forgotten the importance of the gifts, like electrons and electrolytes, that Mother Earth gives us to increase our wellness. Soil, often overlooked and underestimated, is truly the foundation upon which life on land depends. By taking care of the soil, we're taking care of our communities, bodies, and cells in many ways. Soil is responsible for:

+ **Nutrient Recycling:** Soil is like a treasure chest of nutrients that plants need to grow. When plants and animals die, their remains decompose into the soil, releasing important nutrients and electrolytes like nitrogen, phosphorus, and potassium. These nutrients are then taken up by plants, forming the base of the food chain.

+ **Plant Growth:** Soil gives plants a place to put down roots and grow. It provides plants with water, nutrients, and a sturdy foundation. Healthy soil helps plants thrive, which in turn provides habitat and food for humans and animals.

+ **Water Management:** Soil acts like a sponge, soaking up water when it rains and slowly releasing it to plants over time. This helps recharge groundwater and keeps streams flowing, even during dry spells. Soil also prevents floods by absorbing excess water.

+ **Sustaining Life:** Soil is teeming with life, from tiny bacteria to earthworms. These organisms break down organic matter, recycle nutrients, and help plants grow. Some even form partnerships with plants, providing them with nutrients in exchange for sugars.

+ **Providing Cultural and Economic Value:** Throughout history, soil has been essential for human survival. It's where we grow our food, build our homes, and find resources for medicine and industry. Today, the soil continues to support agriculture and economies around the world.

In short, soil is much more than just dirt. Eating and taking in nutrients is something we all do daily, but we don't often think about how those nutrients got into the food in the first place.

We've learned that plants contain most of the nutrients your cells need, including electrolytes and other minerals. The nutrients then move into your body and cells when you eat the plants or when you eat animals that have eaten them. But where do the plants get the nutrients that they give to you? Are they all in the tiny seed they sprouted from? Nope. The seed contained the nutrients needed to start plant life, but to grow and develop, the plant gathered nutrients from the soil.

The process that gives the soil these valuable nutrients starts with the trillions of microorganisms that live in the soil, including bacteria, fungi, and protozoa. They are the workers that decompose dead plant material, releasing nutrients into the soil in forms that plants can absorb. These nutrients are then absorbed from the soil through the plant's root systems, providing plants with the energy and essential elements needed for their own growth and metabolism, as well as energy and nutrients for your cells when you eat them.

These nutrients are the same ones your appestat is looking for: minerals, vitamins, carbohydrates, fats, proteins, and fiber, as well as water. When plants get proper nutrition, you in turn get proper nutrition when you eat them. Nutrient-rich plants supply your cells and body with what they need for optimal health, support your body's physiological processes, secure your cells and reduce the risk of chronic disease, and improve signals across your body.

Earth Health Equals Your Health

In the simplest terms, you are what you eat, and what you eat comes from the ground. If not for healthy soil, you would not have energy or be able to achieve wellness. The earth keeps itself healthy by recycling dead plant matter to nourish the next crop of plants. It's been doing this for centuries, without the help of a gardener, in the massive forests and fields gracing the earth.

On my homestead, I have a large garden that is overflowing with fruits and vegetables. When people tour the garden, they ask what fertilizer I use to help my tomato plants grow eight feet tall and my broccoli plants spread as wide as arms can reach. They ooh and aah over yellow raspberries as large as a thumb and snow pea pods as long as their hands. Expecting revolutionary fertility secrets, they are all surprised to find that the only fertilizer I use is the same one the forests use: compost, a mixture of decaying plant matter that returns nutrients back to the earth to be reused. This seems so simple, but a combination of changes in food production and handling over the last century has led humans away from natural ways of working with the soil, threatening the earth's ability to support and sustain us.

As humans, we are in a partnership with the earth and her soil. After all, they provide us with nutrient-rich plants to eat as food. The earth and nature must take tiny little seeds and turn them into semitruck-loads of food for us. Honestly, this is miraculous.

What is humanity's part to play in this partnership? Humans must help the soil thrive. We must provide it with nutrients so it can continue to feed the plants that feed us. Unfortunately, as food production demands have increased, human stewardship of the land has suffered. One of the most enduring examples of this poor stewardship is the Dust Bowl of the 1930s, one of the most tragic eras in U.S. agricultural history. At that time, the Great Plains were a seemingly endless sea of grasses stretching as far as the eye could see. To encourage Americans to settle the vast western states, a series of laws called Homestead Acts were passed that granted families land in the Great Plains. Thousands moved west, even though many of them had never farmed before. Homesteaders plowed up the native grasslands, some as tall as six feet high, to make way for crops like wheat, corn, and cotton. In doing so, they transformed complex ecosystems full of grasses, flowers, and natural windbreaks into crop fields growing just one or a few kinds of plants. The homesteaders also used blocks of the thick grasses and the attached soil to make sod huts, leaving the soil underneath naked and exposed. Without the protection of the grasses, the exposed soil would dry out within a day.

When World War I began, the European demand for American crops increased, so homesteaders plowed even more land. They raced to modernize agricultural practices and make as much money off the land as possible. But when the U.S. stock market crashed in 1929 and the Great Depression hit, grain prices dropped severely. Desperate for enough money to survive, the new farmers plowed even more land. But in the early 1930s, there was a devastating drought. Rainfall dwindled, temperatures soared, and the parched earth cracked under the relentless sun. As crops withered and livestock perished, desperation set in among farmers already struggling to make ends meet. The once-sturdy prairie sod, which had evolved over millennia to withstand the harsh environmental conditions of the Great Plains, was now gone. Without the deep-rooted grasses anchoring the soil and its moisture in place, the soil became vulnerable to erosion.

This phenomenon has been called the Dust Bowl for a reason. The wind began to pick up the bare soil, blowing layers of dust onto livestock, roads, homes, and cars, even reaching all the way to New York City, where the dust coated the side of the Statue of Liberty and the decks of ships in New York Harbor. On April 14, 1935, later called "Black Sunday," the horrors of the Dust Bowl peaked. A massive dust storm fueled by high winds and drought-dried soil swept across the Great Plains, enveloping the landscape in a dense cloud of thick, choking dust. The sky turned black as night and visibility plummeted to near zero, plunging communities into darkness in the middle of the day. The dust killed crops, livestock, people, and dreams. Farmers had plowed up the roots that once secured their land, and in so doing they destroyed their livelihoods.

You would think humankind would learn from that tragic era, but we didn't. Today, people are experiencing what I call a "nutritional dust bowl." Explosive population growth in the last century has not been followed by a growth in farmers. In fact, the opposite has occurred. Annual farm survey data dating back to 1950 shows a clear trend of fewer farms and fewer acres used for agriculture. Since 1950, the number of farms has decreased by 3.75 million (66 percent) and the number of acres being farmed decreased by 323 million (27 percent). There is only one farmer for every 350 people in the U.S. That's a difficult ratio to manage for any farm and farmer. To make sure they stay afloat, farmers must squeeze every last bushel out of their soil. This has pitted your nutrition against the economics of agriculture, which is a lose-lose battle.[210]

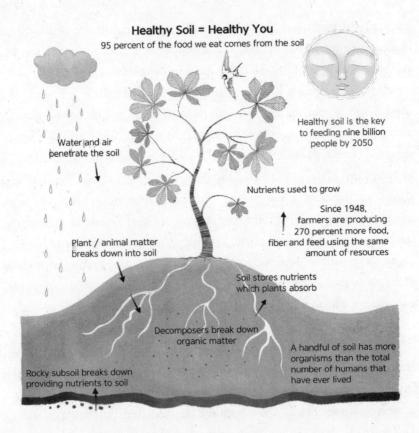

Healthy Soil = Healthy You
95 percent of the food we eat comes from the soil

Healthy soil is the key to feeding nine billion people by 2050

Water and air penetrate the soil

Nutrients used to grow

Since 1948, farmers are producing 270 percent more food, fiber and feed using the same amount of resources

Plant / animal matter breaks down into soil

Soil stores nutrients which plants absorb

Decomposers break down organic matter

A handful of soil has more organisms than the total number of humans that have ever lived

Rocky subsoil breaks down providing nutrients to soil

The Invisible Deficiency

To keep up with the growing demand for food, farmers have made significant changes to the way their farms operate. The rise of industrial agriculture in the twentieth century revolutionized food production, processing, and distribution. Today, vast fields are dedicated to monocropping, where single crops like wheat, corn, and soybeans are grown extensively. These crops are engineered for high yields, with size, growth rate, and pest resistance prioritized above nutritional value. Because the same crop is grown repeatedly on the same land, monocropping depletes the soil of specific nutrients. This results in crops that lack the nutritional content found in older, more diverse varieties.[211] Additionally, monocrops are more susceptible to pests and diseases, leading farmers with monocrops to become increasingly reliant on pesticides and herbicides. These chemicals disrupt the soil microbiome, further diminishing its ability to produce plants that are rich in nutrients.

The relentless push for higher yields has also led to the introduction of genetically modified organisms (GMOs), which were intended to improve efficiency but have also disrupted the ecosystems they're introduced into. GMOs contribute to the development of "super" pests and weeds that have become resistant to pesticides and herbicides. This can lead to them spreading unchecked. Industrialized agriculture practices like these aim to maximize food production on shrinking farmland. While these practices have increased food quantity, they have compromised the nutritional quality and health of the soil.[212] The soil, once a vibrant wellspring of nutritional value, is now struggling to provide the essential nutrients, electrons, and electrolytes that healthy crops—and human cells—need.

In order to address this problem, commercial farming has come to rely heavily on chemical fertilizers to boost crop yields. Soil scientists have learned that plants will grow green and tall with three essential nutrients: nitrogen (N), phosphorus (P), and potassium (K). These chemical heavyweights, combined as fertilizer, boost crop yields and ensure that our staple foods—corn, wheat, and soy—are easy to grow and transport. However, though these fertilizers may increase plant growth, they do not feed the soil. And when the soil is poor in nutrients, the plants grown in it are also poor in nutrients. This creates a food supply that appears healthy but lacks essential electrons, electrolytes, and other nutrients your body and cells need from the earth.

Grocery shelves and even many bellies are overflowing, yet those same bodies are starving for the nutrients that will give their cells the energy potential that they really need. In the United States, government farm subsidies help make corn, soy, and wheat supremely affordable, so they dominate the food supply. This has given rise to endless rows of ultra-cheap, processed foods, which are often blamed for the nation's ballooning obesity rates and related health woes, like heart disease, cancer, and diabetes. Corn, transformed into high-fructose corn syrup, sneaks into countless products, sweetening your food while souring your health by contributing to weight gain, spiking blood sugar levels, increasing the risk of insulin resistance, and promoting inflammation. Over time, these effects can lead to a higher risk of chronic diseases like diabetes, heart disease, and fatty liver disease.[213, 214] But here's the real kicker: as crops have been bred to produce more, produce faster, and to withstand traveling long distances, they have become mere shadows of their nutrient-rich ancestors. To make sure your cells stay well, the way food is grown needs to be changed.

Where Do We Go from Here?

The earth and the things harvested from her soil have the potential to supply the energy your cells need and to save your health. The further away you get from the earth, the easier it becomes to forget that the plants that grow in the earth's soil are the source of the energy and nutrients in your food. Every bite you take of those plants, every step you take with your feet directly connected to the earth, and every dollar you spend on food from small, organic farms has the potential to change both your health and the world. Sustainable practices like crop rotation, organic farming, and regenerative agriculture are gaining ground, and they promise to replenish the soil and the plants that grow from it with the crucial elements they've been missing. These changes help to reconnect humankind with the earth.

The food you eat can be rich in nutrients and give you boundless energy. This isn't just about growing food or harvesting electrons or electrolytes; this is about living well.

Chapter 7
Keyhole Concepts

....

+ Electrons that you harvest from the soil are a kind of non-pharmaceutical therapy that can restore energy to your cells and body. Vitamin G, as it has been called, is free, easy to implement,

and improves quality of living by adding more electrons to your
cells and body.

✦ The diverse array of nutrients your cells and body need to stay well
can only be obtained from plant-based foods that have been grown
in nutrient-rich soil.

✦ Soil itself is a living entity and needs to be cultivated and sustained
so that the food it produces can continue to provide people with the
energy and food that they need to have healthy cells.

✦ Processed foods are high in calories and low in the nutrients that
you need to help your cells stay well.

✦ All the products discussed in this chapter can be found at
www.resources.livingwellbook.com.

CHAPTER 8

Air

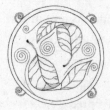

Every cell in your body depends on oxygen to survive. Oxygen, often taken for granted, can help you stay well and act as powerful medicine. Just like the earth, oxygen is essential for life. It can help prevent and treat inflammation, chronic diseases, poor focus, ADHD, congenital anomalies, dementia, headaches, anxiety, depression, and chronic fatigue. The best part? Everyone has access to it, it's all around us, and it's absolutely free! Oxygen plays many roles in your body, including fueling energy and ATP production, reducing inflammation, and even preventing cancer. In fact, the average person needs about one cup of oxygen per minute to sustain essential functions like heart, brain, and immune system activity while at rest, and during strenuous activity, this demand skyrockets to nearly two gallons of oxygen per minute.[215]

When your cells and body get enough oxygen, you can stay well and heal rapidly. However, there are three common obstacles to getting enough oxygen for cellular health: airway blockages or obstructions, air pollution, and lack of nutrients that cells require to utilize oxygen properly. Let's learn how to get as much of this life-giving element as your cells need!

Nutritional science studies how essential nutrients like proteins, carbohydrates, and fats are processed in the body to maintain health, support growth, and prevent disease. However, nutritional science often overlooks two other critical substances: oxygen/air and water. Are these elements actually nutrients? Because life is not possible without them, oxygen/air and water are considered nutrients and medicines in the Cell Well model. Oxygen can correct a host of ailments such as heart failure, respiratory infections, trauma and medical emergencies, sleep apnea, headaches, anemia, wounds, and more. It is literally the most crucial substance for living organisms. You can survive three weeks without food, three days without water, but only three minutes without air. You require oxygen for the healthy functioning of every organ and tissue in your body.

Oxygen's Journey to the Cells

How do you get that oxygen to your cells? The answer lies in your body's respiratory system (nose, windpipe, diaphragm, breathing muscles, and lungs). The respiratory system's main job is to bring fresh air that contains oxygen into the body and move waste gas out. When you breathe in, millions of miniature air sacs in your lungs called alveoli fill with oxygen-rich air. The oxygen then moves into your blood by passing through the very thin walls of the air sacs and into tiny blood vessels within the lungs called capillaries. Just like taxis lined up outside the airport waiting to take travelers to their next destination, red blood cells squeeze through narrow capillaries in a single file line, and a protein called hemoglobin in each cell readies itself to pick up the oxygen. Once the oxygen has been picked up, these newly oxygenated red blood cells travel in the blood vessels from the lungs to the left side of your heart, where they are pumped out and around your entire body. When each oxygenated red blood cell arrives at its destination cell, it exchanges the oxygen it is carrying for carbon dioxide, a waste gas. The carbon dioxide–filled red blood cells then travel through the veins back to the right side of your heart. This side of the heart pumps blood back to your lungs, where the carbon dioxide is released from the blood into the air sacs to be breathed out. With your next inhale, oxygen is again picked up by your blood and the journey begins again. This incredibly efficient, vital process, known as gas exchange, is managed by your lungs and respiratory system without you even having to think about it.[216]

Oxygen is essential for your body because it:

+ is a key ingredient in the creation of energy in every cell.[217]
+ strengthens the immune system, building resistance to infections and preventing microbes from thriving.[218]
+ eliminates waste gases from the body.[219]
+ assists in digestion, especially of fats and carbohydrates.[220]
+ enables your body to "burn" fat more effectively.[221]
+ neutralizes lactic acid, which builds up in hard-working muscles.[222]
+ helps tissues heal faster and reduces inflammation.[223]

Oxygen Is Necessary for Energy Production

When a cell needs oxygen, this gas is allowed through the secure cell wall and supplied to the mitochondria, the cell's power plant. When there is an adequate supply of oxygen, mitochondria can generate thirty-six molecules of ATP per cycle of energy production. However, if oxygen levels are low, a less efficient process must be used, and only two ATP molecules are produced per cycle. When oxygen is low, energy production is inefficient, and the resulting lack of sufficient energy in your cells puts strain on your body. This explains why you breathe so hard during intense exercise: the more energy your body needs, the more oxygen your cells demand. While cells can survive with low oxygen levels and minimal ATP production, this can lead to fatigue and disorders including immune over- or under-activity, cancer, heart disease, and other degenerative processes associated with aging. When your cells don't get enough oxygen, they are literally slowly dying. Ensuring a steady supply of oxygen keeps your cells, and you, going strong.

Sam Wasn't Living Well

When I first saw Sam as a patient, I was struck by how old he looked for his thirty-one years. He and his wife Alicia had four young, energetic kids, which might have explained some of his fatigue, but certainly not all of it. Sam's mother-in-law had suggested he see me, hoping there was a dental infection or issue that could explain his exhaustion. As soon as I looked into his mouth, I knew Sam's lack of energy wasn't due to an infection; it was an oxygen problem. Sam's smile revealed a mouthful of jumbled teeth, all competing for space in a jaw that was much too small for them. The roof of his mouth was narrow, leading to crowded teeth and a strained lower jaw. His tongue was "tied" to the floor of his mouth, leaving it nowhere to go but back into his windpipe day and night. Whether due to genetics, environmental factors, or a combination of both, Sam's facial development had left him with virtually no room to breathe.

During the day, Sam struggled to get enough air to generate the energy needed for basic tasks. At night, his breathing issues made it impossible for him to sleep deeply, causing him to toss and turn and never feel fully rested. As I explained my findings, Sam and Alicia quietly began to cry. Sam's difficulties with waking up on time had cost him several jobs, and even when he was employed, he couldn't work as quickly as he needed to. At home, he spent most of his time in bed, unable to help Alicia with the kids or the household chores. Desperate and emotional, Alicia asked if there were any solutions. I explained how Sam could wear a specialized mouth appliance, like a retainer, to widen the roof of his mouth and the base of his nose. This, along with releasing his tied-down tongue with a simple laser procedure, would create more room in his mouth and airway for air to flow to his lungs. As Sam and Alicia listened, tears came again as they felt hope for the first time in a long time.

Oxygen's Connection to Inflammation

When cells have enough oxygen, not only do they generate the energy you need, but they also grow, thrive, reproduce, and die when and how they need to. However, when oxygen levels in your cells drop, your body's defense system sounds an alarm, which in turn triggers inflammation. Inflammation can be caused by:

1. **Cell Stress:** Oxygen deprivation stresses cells, leading to oxidative damage to DNA, proteins, and lipids, and triggering inflammation. Prolonged cell stress can cause mutations, disrupt cell functions, and contribute to chronic health issues.[224]

2. **Immune Activation:** When cells don't have enough oxygen, special proteins called hypoxia-inducible factors switch on genes that cause inflammation, which attracts immune cells that further increase inflammation.[225]

3. **Waste Production:** Low cellular oxygen can cause a buildup of the waste product lactic acid. Accumulation of lactic acid can contribute to increased inflammation and tissue damage.[226]

4. **Leaky Blood Vessels:** Low oxygen can make the cells lining your blood vessels more permeable or porous, allowing immune cells to pass through where they normally wouldn't, which can start an inflammatory response.[227]

Although inflammation can be helpful in signaling your body to flood an injured or infected site with plasma and white blood cells, inflammation that has become chronic can cause harm. In fact, when cells are exposed to low oxygen levels (a condition known as hypoxia) for a prolonged period, they start activating certain proteins called *hypoxia-inducible factors* (HIFs). These HIFs act like switches, turning on genes that help cells survive in low-oxygen conditions. However, these same genes can also make the cells start behaving abnormally.

Instead of following normal growth and division rules, hypoxic cells may begin to divide more quickly and ignore signals to stop growing. This is because HIFs can activate genes that promote rapid cell division and create new blood vessels, helping to feed the growing cell mass. Over time, this uncontrolled cell growth can lead to the formation of tumors, ultimately increasing the risk of cancer.[228]

Additionally, low oxygen levels can throw your immune system off balance. An immune system weakened by lack of oxygen is like an army sent into battle without proper gear: it's not as effective at its protective job, including stopping cancer growth. This weakened immune response gives cancer cells an opportunity to thrive and multiply. Basically, low oxygen paired with the resulting inflammation creates a cozy environment for cancer cells to flourish. It provides them with the perfect conditions to grow rapidly, evade the immune system, and even spread to other parts of the body, a process known as metastasis.[229]

Understanding Inflammation

Chronic inflammation can lead not only to cancer, but also to other immune-system-gone-awry conditions like insulin resistance, diabetes, and heart disease.[230] What leads to overzealous immune responses and chronic inflammation? Several factors can contribute:

Supply

+ **Processed Foods:** Diets high in processed foods such as cookies, cakes, and candies; chips, crackers, and flavored popcorn; processed meats like hot dogs, sausages, and deli meats; fast food items like burgers, fries, and fried chicken; and convenience foods such as frozen meals, instant noodles, and canned soups can all lead to inflammation in the cells and body.[231]

+ **Unhealthy Fats:** Fats that can promote inflammation in the body include trans fats used in many processed and fried foods, saturated fats in fatty meats, full-fat dairy products, some processed foods like baked goods and snacks, and omega-6 fatty acids found in vegetable oils like soybean oil and corn oil.[232]

Support

+ **Autoimmune Disorders:** This misguided immune response, in which the body's immune system attacks its own cells and tissues, can lead to inflammation, tissue damage, and dysfunction of affected organs or systems.[233]
+ **Lack of Exercise:** Physical inactivity leads to reduced blood flow and oxygen delivery to tissues, contributing to cellular stress.[234]
+ **Aging:** Chronic low-grade inflammation, often dubbed "inflammaging," is a common occurrence as individuals age. This state of persistent mild inflammation is associated with various age-related diseases and health issues.[235]

Secure

+ **Ongoing Infection:** Viruses like hepatitis B or C and bacterial infections like tuberculosis can live in the body for a long time, keeping the immune system continuously engaged.[236]
+ **Environmental Toxins:** Exposure to environmental pollutants, such as air pollution, pesticides, and heavy metals, can trigger and contribute to chronic inflammation over time.[237]

Signal

+ **Obesity:** Fat cells, especially visceral fat (fat around the organs), send cytokine warning signals. The more cells there are, the more pronounced the reaction can become.[238]

✦ **Chronic Stress:** Prolonged stress leads to prolonged signaling from hormones like cortisol, which can dysregulate the immune system, leading to chronic inflammation.[239]

Inflammation lies at the heart of a growing health crisis, contributing to the rise of chronic diseases that plague millions worldwide. Shockingly, statistics reveal that three out of five deaths globally are connected to chronic inflammatory conditions like stroke, respiratory diseases, heart ailments, cancer, obesity, and diabetes.[240]

Oxygen is a key player in combating this inflammation.

Why Your Cells Can't Get Enough Oxygen

As you may remember, there are three major factors that can make getting enough oxygen difficult: airway blockages, air pollution, and a lack of the nutrients that cells require to utilize oxygen properly. First, let's talk about airway blockages.

Airway blockages can arise from various causes, such as a stubborn sinus infection, a sports-related injury to the nose, or developmental issues affecting the mouth and nose structure. All these causes lead to one common complaint I hear every day in my dental practice: sleep troubles. A staggering number of patients across the globe share difficulties with falling asleep, early awakenings, incessant tossing and turning, and snoring or teeth grinding. This silent epidemic of sleep disorders is on the rise. According to recent data, fifty to seventy million Americans have sleep disorders, and one in three adults do not get the recommended amount of uninterrupted sleep. In fact, a meta-analysis of studies found that 55.64 percent of people have poor sleep quality, and 33.32 percent of students experience excessive sleepiness during the day.[241] Many of these problems can be attributed to inadequate air and oxygen supply.

Let's take a closer look at some common signs of an airway blockage or sleep disorder.

Signs of Airway Blockage

+ Snoring
+ Pauses in breathing, or gasping or choking during sleep
+ Waking at night to go to the bathroom
+ Difficulty falling asleep
+ Waking frequently or too early and feeling unable to go back to sleep
+ Grinding or clenching your teeth
+ Acid reflux making your throat feel sore at night or in the morning

Symptoms During the Day

+ Daytime exhaustion
+ Difficulty concentrating (ADHD symptoms)
+ Morning headaches
+ Dark circles under your eyes
+ Sore muscles in your jaw and face
+ Bedwetting in children

Signs in Your Mouth

+ Extra growths of bone on the jawbone next to the tongue, called tori
+ Worn-out or flattened teeth
+ Indentations or "scallops" around the outside of your tongue
+ Dry mouth or throat upon waking
+ Tooth decay
+ Enlarged tonsils

If you experience any of these symptoms, it's time to take steps to increase your airflow—and reclaim your sleep.

Carol Couldn't Breathe

Carol, a new patient, came to my practice because she had some swelling under her nose and her front teeth were a little loose. Both of those teeth had received root canals years ago, and she wondered if that could be the problem. But when I took a cone beam CT scan, I found more than either Carol or I had expected. The root canals had gotten reinfected, and the infection had destroyed a significant amount of the jawbone around the tooth roots, explaining why the teeth were loose. From the extent of the bone loss, it was apparent the infection had been there for a very long time. Why hadn't Carol known about it?

Carol had gotten the root canals on her two front teeth after a cheerleading accident in middle school. Her parents had been saving money so she could have braces, but the root canals used up her braces fund, so her teeth stayed crowded. In college, the teeth with the root canals started to darken, so Carol had crowns made to cover them so they would look better. In the decades that followed, Carol's teeth with root canals didn't hurt because the nerve had been removed, but she said they never "felt right." Carol's immune system had been efficiently cleaning up the area, and she hadn't experienced any symptoms until now.

Because of the longstanding bone loss, there was no longer enough bone to hold her front teeth in place, and both had to be removed. Understandably, Carol was upset! My team reassured her that we would be able to replace the teeth with ceramic dental implants, and at the end of the treatment, her smile would be better than ever. Carol agreed to have the teeth removed and the infection cleaned out, and slowly her mouth started to heal.

During a follow-up visit, I asked Carol how she was feeling. She offhandedly mentioned that she must have been tired after the surgery because she had been sleeping so deeply that she wasn't even snoring. Seeing her worn-out and crowded teeth, the scallop-shaped indentations on the side of her tongue, and the big extra growth of bone under her tongue, I recommended she have a sleep study done. She insisted she slept as well as anyone else but agreed. When her results came back, Carol and I found that she had severe sleep apnea. The only medical problem Carol had noted in her medical history survey was heart problems, but as we talked, we both realized she was not as well as her medical history suggested.

She had struggled for decades to go to sleep at night and had tried every sleep hack the internet could provide: melatonin, no screens before bed, hot baths in the evening, a magnesium-rich drink at bedtime, and more. Desperate, she finally resorted to medicating with a pharmaceutical sleep aid. Carol's snoring had worsened over the years, and even though her husband started the night in her bed, she frequently woke to him sleeping in another room. She was groggy and moody in the morning, and she frequently woke up with a headache. Even when Carol felt like she had slept well, in truth she still spent the hours tossing and turning. Everyone in the family knew not to talk to Carol until she had finished one or two cups of coffee, and they laughed when she couldn't remember simple things like her granddaughter's birthday or where she had left her keys. Thinking her symptoms were normal parts of life and aging, Carol had a logical explanation for everything she was experiencing, and no reason to suspect sleep apnea.

The big wake-up call came after Carol had chest pains one evening. She brushed them off for hours until she couldn't breathe without grimacing. Carol's husband rushed her to the ER, where the doctors hooked her up to a room full of sensors and monitors and poked and prodded until an anxious-looking resident told her she had experienced a mild heart attack. Fortunately, her husband's fast action and the doctor's clot-busting drugs helped her have a smooth recovery with few lasting symptoms. After her heart attack, Carol stopped taking the pharmaceutical sleep aid and spent many hours every night wide awake. Until after her dental surgery.

As Carol and I sifted through her medical and dental history, we started to put together some very important clues. Carol realized her sleeping problems started in high school after the cheerleading accident, subsequent root canals, and crowded teeth. As the years passed, her sleeping problems worsened, along with her acid reflux, food sensitivities, and high blood pressure. All these symptoms, including the heart attack, were her cells screaming for her to pay attention. Remember, symptoms are your body's warning signs that something is wrong at the cellular level. Could Carol's heart and digestion problems really have stemmed from her poor sleep all along? And could her sleep have been affected by the infected teeth and crowding in her mouth? Carol shook her head in disbelief as we worked our way back through her history.

The arrangement and health of your teeth affect everything else in your mouth. When your teeth are crowded and there is too little room in your mouth, your tissues, tonsils, and muscles spill back into the areas you use to breathe, blocking airflow and reducing the amount of oxygen you are getting day and night. This is worse at night because when you lie down, all the crowded tissues fall even further back, interfering with the airflow or even stopping it completely. This phenomenon is called obstructive sleep apnea. This is exactly what happened to Carol. Her small, crowded mouth had left her too little room to breathe. Her infections compounded the problem because the inflammation in her mouth led to swelling in the tissues in the mouth and the throat, further blocking her airflow.

During sleep apnea, the body's emergency "fight-or-flight" response system is activated every time breathing is interrupted. Carol's body perceived these interruptions as life-threatening events, prompting an emergency response that looks like this:

1. When the airway becomes partially or completely blocked, blood oxygen levels drop. The brain detects this drop through sensors in the blood vessels.

2. The brain signals your adrenal glands to release stress hormones like adrenaline, which increase heart rate and blood pressure to quickly restore oxygen levels.

3. The brain also triggers a brief awakening or arousal to reopen the airway—often so brief that the person is not aware of the disruption to their sleep cycle.

4. This brief waking cues muscles to force the airway open, which is often accompanied by grinding and clenching teeth.

5. When the muscles relax again, it's only a matter of time before the airflow is reobstructed and the cycle begins again.

Repeated activation of this response throughout the night prevents deep, restorative sleep. It also causes a continual release of stress hormones, which can lead to high blood pressure, increased risk of heart attack and stroke, systemic infection, and metabolic disorders like diabetes and thyroid problems.[242]

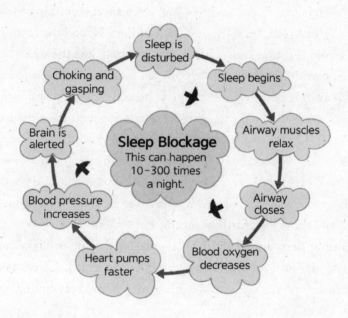

Carol was fighting for her life night after night. After relenting and taking medications, she was no longer "awake" at night, but she wasn't really asleep either. The snoring, tossing and turning, and teeth clenching all prevented her from entering deep sleep mode, when the brain "backs up" memories, rebuilds cells, and reboots its internal systems. Good-quality sleep is so crucial that without it, your risk of dementia and Alzheimer's increases by 70 percent and your life expectancy decreases by 20 percent. After I explained these things to Carol, her struggles with memory, digestive issues, and fatigue all made sense, and she even realized that her sleep apnea could have been a primary factor in the heart attack she was lucky to survive. Low oxygen, high blood pressure, and increased inflammation can cause heart disease, arrhythmia, and heart attacks or failure, just like Carol experienced.

Side Effects of Sleep Apnea

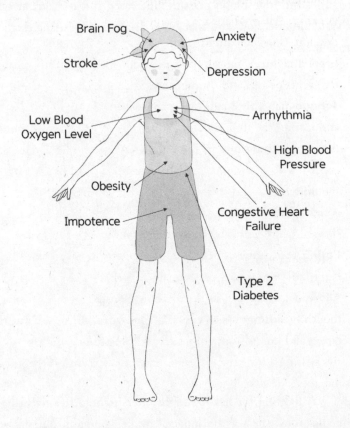

Obstructive sleep apnea or OSA is surprisingly common, affecting nearly 34 percent of men and 17 percent of women worldwide.[243] In people whose hearts, lungs, and vessels are already unwell, the incidence jumps to as high as 80 percent. Despite these high numbers, airflow and sleep disturbances are often underrecognized, underdiagnosed, and left untreated.[244] This is an especially deadly oversight since cardiovascular disease, like the heart attack Carol had, is the number one cause of death globally and the cause of one out of every three deaths in the United States.[245]

Several factors throughout life may lead to your airway becoming obstructed. Let's learn more about a few of them.

During Infancy and Childhood

+ **Prolonged bottle feeding, pacifier use, sippy cup use, or thumb sucking:** All of these may change the way the mouth and face develop. (Prolonged means longer than typical, i.e., bottle feeding beyond eighteen months of age, pacifier or sippy cup use beyond two years of age, and thumb sucking at any age.)

+ **Tongue-tie:** This condition occurs when the small band of tissue connecting the underside of the tongue to the floor of the mouth is too tight and prevents the tongue from reaching the roof of the mouth. Without tongue pressure against the roof of the mouth, the mouth and jaw can't form correctly.

+ **A small mouth:** This can be either developmental or due to orthodontic treatment focused on straight teeth at the expense of room for air.

+ **Eating too many processed, soft, easy-to-digest foods:** This can hinder proper muscle and jaw growth.

+ **Allergies:** These can lead to swollen tonsils, a blocked nose, and mouth breathing, which causes air to bypass the nose's natural filtering and humidifying functions, leading to dry mouth, increased risk of infections, poor oxygen exchange, and potential dental issues like tooth decay and gum disease.

During Adult Years

+ **Allergies or injuries to the nose:** These can lead to blocked nasal passages and mouth breathing.

+ **Infection in the head and neck:** It is possible that this can be caused by an infected tooth or infection in the area of the jawbone area where a tooth was removed.

+ **Having a large neck or excess weight in the neck area:** This increases the amount of tissue that can potentially block the airway.

+ **Eating packaged, processed foods:** This can cause inflammation in the cells and body, which in turns causes swelling in the airway.

For years, I wondered why patients like Carol, when asked, said they didn't have problems sleeping. But Carol had adapted, and because she didn't know what a good night's sleep felt like, she didn't know what she was missing. Because sleep is an automatic body process, it isn't something you should have to consciously work for. You should expect to be able to just lie down at night and sleep! But if your body must choose getting enough air over sleeping, the need for air will win every time, and you won't sleep.

Pay attention to the quality of your sleep, because poor sleep is one of the indicators that your cells need help. To determine if you are getting too little air and are at risk for these serious health problems, take the Sleeping Well Assessment below.

Sleeping Well Assessment

Date of Assessment:

Physical Symptoms:

Place a checkmark next to symptoms you experience at least a few times per week.	**Yes**
Do you often feel excessively sleepy during the day, even after a full night's sleep?	_____
Do you struggle to stay awake while driving or during other activities?	_____
Does your bed partner or a family member complain about your loud snoring?	_____
Has anyone noticed that you stop breathing or gasp for air during sleep?	_____
Does your bed partner notice you tossing and turning frequently during sleep?	_____
Does your bed partner notice you waking up frequently during the night?	_____

Do you wake one to two times a week with headaches in the morning? _____

Do you often wake up with a dry mouth or sore throat? _____

Do you wake up two or more times during the night to urinate? _____

Do you have trouble concentrating during the day? _____

Have you experienced mood swings or irritability? _____

Have you noticed a decrease in your sex drive? _____

Do you have difficulty remembering things or experience memory lapses? _____

Do you find it challenging to solve problems or make decisions? _____

Have you experienced symptoms of depression or anxiety? _____

Do you feel less motivated to engage in activities you used to enjoy? _____

Is the measurement around your neck greater than 17 inches (43 cm) if you are a man, or 16 inches (41 cm) if you are a woman? _____

Do you have crowded teeth? _____

Does your chin appear to be set back or receding? _____

Have you ever been diagnosed with enlarged tonsils or adenoids? _____

Total Score (out of 20): _____

This checklist can serve as a screening tool for assessing the likelihood of obstructive sleep apnea or sleep-disordered breathing.

Assessment Tally: How many boxes did you check?

1–4: Practice Living Well Fall/Air Recommendations for better sleep.

4–7: Practice Living Well Fall/Air and Spring/Plants Recommendations, and consider visiting a sleep-focused dentist or doctor for a sleep test.

7+: Visit a sleep-focused dentist or doctor to have a sleep test performed.

(For print and digital versions of this screening, go to www.resources.livingwellbook.com.)

Air Pollution Is a Problem

Correcting any blockages that prevent air from reaching your lungs is the starting point for getting enough oxygen to your cells. But the quality of the air you breathe is also very important. Air pollution is a major contributor to oxygen deficiency today.

I live in a valley surrounded by tall mountains, and in the dark days of winter, we often get inversions, which is when warm air is trapped close to the ground by a layer of cooler air above it. This layer acts like a lid, preventing the warm air near the surface from rising and trapping pollutants close to the ground. When this happens, the air is so yellow and thick you can see and almost taste it. The yellow air hangs in the valley until a storm comes in and washes it away. This inversion leads to poor air quality, which leads to increased health risks.

Pollutants in the air, especially in urban areas or areas with heavy industrial activity, can displace oxygen molecules in the air, reducing the amount of oxygen available for breathing. These pollutants also damage the lungs, potentially leading to asthma, chronic obstructive pulmonary disease (COPD), and other respiratory illnesses that affect the lungs' ability to take in oxygen effectively. Some of the tiniest molecules of pollutants can even penetrate deep into the lungs and enter the bloodstream, interfering with your blood's exchange of oxygen and carbon dioxide and leading to oxygen deficiency all the way down to the cellular level.[246]

When you breathe clean air, it contains about 20 percent oxygen. But when there are pollutants like harmful tiny particles from vehicle exhaust, carbon monoxide, ammonia, or heavy metals in the air you're breathing, they affect your wellness in three ways:

1. The pollutants themselves are toxic to your cells and body.

2. When you breathe in air filled with pollutants, you are also breathing in less oxygen, which means too little oxygen gets to your cells. This results in low energy and increased infection, inflammation, and serious disease.

3. These pollutants block out sunlight, which affects plants and their ability to make energy (and produce oxygen) through photosynthesis. When plants' leaves receive less sunlight, less oxygen can be generated and released into the atmosphere. That means less oxygen available for your cells and body to use in the future.[247]

How to Protect Yourself from Outdoor Air Pollution

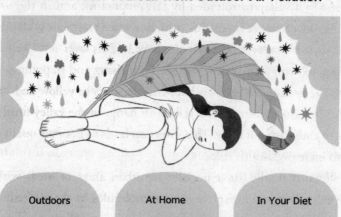

Outdoors	At Home	In Your Diet
Use a face mask	Vacuum often and use ventilation systems	Drink more water
Avoid congested areas	Use air purifiers and clean filters	Eat food rich in Vitamins C and E and omega-3s
Avoid jogging and outdoor activities	Keep windows and doors open	Avoid alcohol and caffeine
Check air quality index in your area	Keep air purifying plants at home	Eat or drink natural decongestants like ginger and green tea

It can be easy to underestimate the importance of maintaining indoor air quality, but breathing clean air is crucial both outdoors and indoors. Even before the COVID-19 pandemic heightened awareness of indoor air quality, poor indoor air was already a risk factor for several of the world's leading causes of death, including heart disease, pneumonia, stroke, diabetes, and lung cancer, and one of the leading risk factors for death globally.[248] Even though many people spend 80–90 percent of their time indoors, there is generally a lack of appreciation and awareness of the significance of the air they breathe inside their homes and other buildings. Unlike outdoor air, the quality of indoor air is not regulated, and indoor air pollution levels are often higher than those outdoors, with concentrations of pollutants sometimes reaching two to five times—and occasionally up to one hundred times—higher than outdoor levels.[249]

The problem of indoor pollution has become even more concerning since the pandemic, as telework and increased indoor time have become more and more common, a trend likely to continue in the future. Numerous studies report strong associations between pollutant contamination in buildings and health problems, particularly allergies.

When you breathe oxygen-deficient air, your body sends you signals such as irritation of the eyes, nose, and throat, headaches, dizziness, and fatigue. In addition to watching for these signals or symptoms, you can purchase a portable air quality monitor to evaluate your air. If you feel that poor air quality is something affecting your cells and health, check out further recommendations at www.livingwellwithdrmichelle.com/book.

Breathing Well Guide

If you've determined that you have a need for cleaner indoor air, and you're ready to take action to find what your cells and body need, you may find yourself overwhelmed by the seemingly dizzying array of options on the market. I've created a Breathing Well Guide to help you sift through these options. This is another "good, better, best" guide that will help you choose the right air filtration option for your home.

But first, let's learn a little more about air filters.

Air Filters

The effectiveness of any given air filter is rated on what is called the "MERV"—or Minimum Efficiency Reporting Value—scale. This is a standardized system used to evaluate and compare the efficiency of air filters in trapping airborne particles of various sizes. The scale rates filters from 1 to 16, with higher numbers indicating filters that can capture smaller particles and a higher percentage of particles overall, thereby providing better air quality.

Here are a few common types of air filters:

✦ **Fiberglass filters:** These are basic, low-cost filters made from layered fiberglass fibers.

✦ **Pleated filters:** Made from polyester or cotton paper folded into pleats, these filters have a greater surface area with which to capture particles.

✦ **High efficiency particulate air (HEPA) filters:** HEPA filters are made of a dense mat of glass fibers which are designed to capture very fine particles.

✦ **Activated carbon filters:** These filters, which contain activated carbon, are excellent at removing odors and potentially harmful chemicals called Volatile Organic Compounds (VOCs). These can be found in household products like paint and cleaning supplies, personal care products like perfume and deodorant, building materials including carpet, and as by-products from factories and refineries. They are often used in combination with other filters for more comprehensive air cleaning, though they are less effective at capturing particulates alone.

Feature/ Criteria	Good	Better	Best
Filter Type	Fiberglass filter	Pleated filter	High efficiency particulate air (HEPA) filter
MERV Rating	1–4	7–12	13–16
Airborne Particle Removal	Large particles (dust, lint, pollen)	Smaller particles (pet dander, mold spores)	Very fine particles (bacteria, smoke, viruses)
Lifespan	1–3 months	3–6 months	6–12 months
Cost	Low ($)	Moderate ($$)	High ($$$)
Suitable For	Basic air quality needs	Homes with pets and allergies	Homes with severe allergies, asthma, or medical conditions

Nutrition for Better Oxygen Utilization

The problems your cells experience from a lack of oxygen in the air you breathe can be magnified if the food you eat doesn't provide the nutrients you need to use it. While specific foods don't directly increase oxygen levels in cells, certain nutrients can optimize oxygen use within the body. Foods that have been heavily processed, cooked, and preserved, as well as high-fat foods like meat, eggs, and dairy products, provide very few of these oxygen-supporting nutrients. This is one of the reasons the Standard American Diet has been linked to a variety of degenerative, inflammatory diseases like heart disease, cancer, and diabetes. Here are some key nutrients and their roles in cellular oxygenation:

Supply

+ **Iron:** Iron is a crucial component of hemoglobin, the protein in red blood cells that binds to oxygen and transports it to cells throughout the body. **Find in:** Leafy greens, legumes, nuts and seeds, quinoa, oats.

✦ **Omega-3 Fatty Acids:** Omega-3 fatty acids reduce inflammation and improve blood flow, ensuring adequate oxygen delivery to cells. **Find in:** Flaxseeds, chia and hemp seeds, Brussels sprouts, walnuts.

Support

✦ **Copper:** Copper is involved in the formation of red blood cells and hemoglobin and facilitates the transfer of oxygen from the bloodstream to cells. **Find in:** Dark chocolate, mushrooms, nuts and seeds, spinach, kale.

✦ **B Vitamins:** B vitamins are essential to the production of red blood cells and hemoglobin and support the efficient utilization of oxygen by cells. **Find in:** Sweet potatoes, avocados, mushrooms, bananas, legumes.

Secure

✦ **Vitamin C:** Vitamin C protects cells from oxidative damage and supports the health of blood vessels, which deliver oxygen to tissues and organs. **Find in:** Bell peppers, tomatoes, citrus fruits, strawberries, kiwi.

Signal

✦ **Vitamin E:** Vitamin E helps maintain cell membranes for optimal cellular function and efficient oxygen transport and utilization. **Find in:** Spinach, mangoes, pumpkins, tomatoes, nuts, seeds.

Ensuring that your cells receive adequate oxygen is fundamental for maintaining wellness and producing the energy your body needs to function. Obstructive sleep apnea and sleep-disordered breathing disrupt the oxygen supply during sleep, leading to numerous health complications. Both outdoor and indoor air pollution further compromise oxygen intake by reducing the amount of oxygen available in the air as well as damaging the respiratory system and impacting effective gas exchange. Additionally, low nutrient levels, particularly deficiencies in iron and vitamins crucial for oxygen transport and utilization, make it even harder to deliver sufficient oxygen to your cells. What can you do to ensure you have enough of the crucial air element for wellness? Take the Sleeping Well Assessment to determine if you need to address an airway obstruction, watch outdoor air quality reports, increase oxygen-supporting nutrients (check out recipes in appendix 1), and, if needed, use the Breathing Well Guide to choose the right indoor air filter to ensure every breath will be full of the oxygen your cells need and free of the things they don't.

By prioritizing air and oxygen, you can power up every cell in your body.

Chapter 8
Keyhole Concepts

....

+ You can survive three weeks without food and three days without water, but only three minutes without air. You require oxygen for the healthy functioning of every organ and tissue in your body.

+ Oxygen can help prevent and treat inflammation, chronic diseases, poor focus, ADHD, developmental issues, dementia, headaches, anxiety, depression, and chronic fatigue. Oxygen can also heal a host of ailments and is literally the most crucial substance for living organisms.

+ Three out of five deaths globally are attributed to chronic inflammatory conditions like stroke, respiratory diseases, heart ailments, cancer, obesity, and diabetes. Oxygen is a key player in combating these conditions.

+ Fifty to seventy million Americans have sleep disorders, many of which are connected to nighttime oxygen deficiency. The Sleeping Well Assessment can point you towards next steps if you are concerned you might be having sleep trouble.

✦ Indoor air pollution levels are often higher than those outdoors. Air filters can help you ensure that the air you're breathing at home is good for your cells.

✦ Foods like nuts and seeds, legumes, leafy greens, sweet potatoes, and some fruits provide nutrients that support your body's ability to utilize oxygen efficiently.

CHAPTER 9

Water

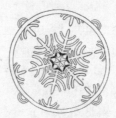

You may daydream about vacationing at the beach or lake, lulled to sleep by the rolling waves. Or maybe you listen to recordings of waves crashing onto the seashore or the gentle gurgling of a stream to fall asleep, or you've felt the intense need for a glass of icy water on a hot summer day.

This strong pull toward water exists because, like air, your life literally depends on it. Sixty percent of your body is water. Water regulates many of your most important metabolic processes, including metabolism, digestion, circulation, and the making of cellular structures and components like proteins and DNA. Water is crucial for health. Water also carries nutrients and other "precious cargo" to every cell in your body. And if your cells get dehydrated, they die. Without water, your cells can't be well, and you literally won't stay alive.

Water is an element that's full of possibilities. The earth's surface is approximately 75 percent water, and you are 60 percent water. Water is changeable; it can be fluid, solid, or gas. It has no shape, taking the form of whatever holds it. Water is the most yielding of all elements, yet it can break down even the hardest rock over time. Water flows in and out of your cells, supporting every essential function.

Water supports your cells in many ways. Brain cells, made up of nearly 80 percent water, are particularly sensitive to hydration levels. Reduction in body water levels can cause decreased mental and physical performance. Blood is about 50 percent water, ferrying nutrients around your body and maintaining your temperature. To keep you at a normal temperature (around 98.6 degrees Fahrenheit, or 37 degrees Celsius), signals from the hypothalamus, a region in the brain that acts as the body's thermostat, direct the flow of blood around the body. When you are too hot, blood moves outward to the skin, widening veins and arteries so that your body can radiate heat into the surrounding air and cool you down. Conversely, when you are cold, blood flows deeper into the body, insulating itself under layers of protective fat and tissue to trap and recycle heat. (Fun fact: this support process is the reason you turn red when you're hot and pale when you're cold!) Another way your body uses water to regulate temperature is through sweat. The evaporation of water via sweat carries heat away from the body many times faster than a breeze on dry skin does, which is also why it's so much harder to stay cool in humid environments.

Water secures your bones and joints, keeping you moving. Water-filled synovial fluid and watery cartilage cushion and lubricate your movements. Together, they absorb impacts, preventing strains, sprains, breaks, and osteoarthritis. Muscles are 75 percent water and bones are 30 percent water.

Water also aids digestion, starting with saliva in the mouth. It produces stomach acid, moves food through the digestive system, and aids its exit through urine and feces. Nearly every chemical reaction in your body uses water.[250]

James, a struggling teenager, learned how crucial water is to his body's systems. After making some questionable life choices, he faced seven weeks in a therapeutic wilderness program. He knew he needed to reset his life. Assigned to a group with similar stories, James quickly learned the schedule: wake at dawn, make a fire, cook dry food mixed with water, then pack for a day on the trail. Each boy had to report their pulse to the trail leaders before hiking. A higher-than-normal pulse rate, or an "off pulse," signaled dehydration. No one in the group could hike until every boy was "on-pulse." James was surprised by how seriously this hydration detector was taken, but it kept him and the other boys healthy while far away from modern medical care. Your body has numerous signals or ways of letting you know what your water levels are, including your heart rate, the color of your urine, your skin's ability to bounce back after stretching, and more.

Cell signaling regulates the amount of water you need to drink, store, and eliminate. Water is stored inside and outside cells in a ratio of two to one, maintained by minerals like chloride, potassium, and sodium. This balance is regulated by hormonal messages from the brain and kidneys. If there's too much of any mineral on one side of the cell membrane, the cell pulls water from the other side to dilute it. This process explains why you get thirsty after eating a salty food like pizza. The brain signals the body to drink more water until the area inside and outside the cells is appropriately diluted for body and cell health. If, responding to the signal, you drink more water than your cells need, the kidneys simply filter that excess and make urine.[251]

Eight Cups of Water a Day?

You've likely heard that you need eight eight-ounce (240-mL) glasses of water each day (the 8x8 rule). That's half a gallon of water (about two liters) per day. This claim is widely accepted and easy to remember, but is it true? Surprisingly, no scientific evidence supports this recommendation.[252] The rule originated from a 1945 U.S. Food and Nutrition Board recommendation of 2.5 liters of daily water intake, rather than actual research. Research suggests this broad recommendation may be too much for some and not enough for others. The actual amount of water that is optimal to drink differs for everyone. You also need to remember that drinking glasses and bottles full of plain water is not the only thing that can hydrate you. Plant foods are an equally important source of water. The following fruits and vegetables are made up largely of water:

+ Cucumber: 95 percent
+ Iceberg lettuce: 95 percent
+ Celery: 95 percent
+ Zucchini: 95 percent
+ Tomatoes: 94 percent
+ Watermelon: 92 percent
+ Strawberries: 91 percent
+ Spinach: 91 percent
+ Cantaloupe: 90 percent
+ Oranges: 86 percent

You also get water from foods like soup, tea, eggs, and gelatin. Other beverages like milk and fruit juice count as well. You could say that the exact amount of water necessary for hydration is "fluid." Every day you lose close to a liter of water from breathing, perspiring, and having bowel movements, but you don't need to follow the eight glasses rule rigidly to stay hydrated. If your cells need more water, your body has a simple signaling mechanism: thirst.[253]

How Water Works

Water is a tiny molecule. It consists of three atoms—two hydrogen and one oxygen—giving it the well-known chemical formula of H_2O. Water's structure allows it to move in and out of cells and carry "cargo" as it goes. Water is also able to exist in three states within the earth's natural temperature ranges: liquid, gas, and solid.

All of earth's water is in motion, moving inside the planet, across its surface, and into the atmosphere above. Water in lakes, rivers, and oceans evaporates with the heat of the sun, plants draw water from the soil and return it to the air, and even volcanoes release water vapor that was locked deep inside rocks. All that water rises and falls back to Earth as rain, snow, sleet, or hail. The water cycle then repeats and repeats, recycling the earth's water. Imagine how far the water you drank traveled to get into your glass; it's been on earth for more than four billion years!

The Water Cycle

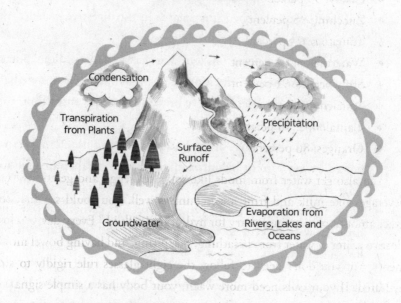

Water's Role in the World and in You

Water has dictated the rise and fall of civilizations. In arid Egypt, the Nile River was a lifeline. The Egyptians built an intricate irrigation system with canals and dikes that controlled the floodwaters and maximized the crops that they could coax out of the land. Control over the Nile and access to its resources often determined a pharaoh's power and influence. Military campaigns were launched to take territories that might threaten Egypt's dominance over the river or give access to additional water resources. Egyptian engineers and rulers understood that their empire's survival depended on water. Waterways provide and transport goods and materials wherever needed.

Your body operates similarly, with internal waterways carrying "cargo" (oxygen, minerals, vitamins, and more) to cells and removing waste. Water brings your cells what they need, supplying them and keeping them well. This cargo is sourced from the other Elements:

+ **Fire:** Water plays a critical role in biochemical reactions, creating space for reactions and participating in electron transfer.
+ **Plants:** Water carries dissolved nutrients like glucose, amino acids, and fatty acids, absorbed from plants in the digestive system, and brings them to cells throughout the body.
+ **Earth:** Water transports ions found in the earth like sodium, potassium, calcium, and magnesium that help maintain electrolyte balance, which is essential for nerve function, muscle contraction, and maintaining fluid balance.
+ **Air:** Through the process of respiration, oxygen molecules are transported by water in the bloodstream to cells, where they are used for cellular energy production.
+ **Water:** Water carries waste products, such as carbon dioxide and urea, away from cells to be excreted from the body through the lungs, kidneys, and other excretory organs.

In the human body, the distribution and regulation of water is controlled by a complex system of hormones and other physiological signals. Hormones and signaling molecules including antidiuretic hormone and aldosterone act like labels on water molecules. Just like the addresses on boxes delivered to your front door, these hormones and signals guide the cargo-filled water molecules to their destinations, instructing them where to go and regulating the speed of delivery. These mechanisms ensure that the body maintains its fluid balance, which is crucial for wellness.

Using Water to Stay Well

The power of water resides in its movement. Water in the natural world is almost always in motion. Waves crash on the beach, streams flow into rivers, and rivers flow into lakes. Rain falls, steam rises, and all this movement creates a powerful release of electrons that your body can use to increase healing in your cells. I learned about this healing power personally when a family friend spiraled into a deep and unshakable depression. In desperation, she moved to the beach where she could soak in electrons from the crashing waves. Her mind and body healed as she recharged her cells.

This isn't an unusual result of being near water. In fact, studies show that people report significantly better mental and overall health when living nearer the coast. How does water bring better health? Water affects many of your senses, and improves mental and overall health in a variety of ways.

- ✦ **Sight:** Blue is associated with feelings of calm and peace.[254] Gazing at the ocean can actually alter your brain waves, inducing a mild meditative state.
- ✦ **Sound:** Hearing the consistent ebb and flow of water calms your brain. The sounds activate your parasympathetic nervous system, which is responsible for slowing you down and allowing you to relax.[255]
- ✦ **Smell:** The scent of the ocean breeze also contributes to your soothed state, due largely to the negative ions in the air that you're breathing in. Negative ions are generated by the movement of water, like waves crashing against the shore, waterfalls, and sea spray. These negatively charged ions have extra electrons to give you and your cells, and they even increase the levels of serotonin in the brain, alleviating symptoms of depression and anxiety.[256]
- ✦ **Touch:** Swimming, soaking in a warm bath, or wading or walking in water can stimulate the release of endorphins, which are natural mood elevators. If you're also touching the earth at the same time, like on a seashore, the water will conduct electrons from the earth to your cells, amping up its grounding effect. Contact with water can also relax muscles and enhance blood circulation.[257]

Source Matters

Water is very good at delivering the cargo that your cells need, but it can also carry toxins and other impurities as well. The water that you drink has likely picked up a lot of unwelcome hitchhikers. Water is one of the most contaminated resources on earth, tainted by additives such as chlorine, fluoride, pesticides, and metals.[258] In fact, a sampling of more than seventy-five thousand sources of water in eighty-nine countries found more than 40 percent of them to be polluted.[259] Toxins you would never knowingly put in your body can sneak in through water.

Luckily, your body has amazing waste- and toxin-removal processes: your lungs remove toxic gases, your digestive tract eliminates dangerous toxins through vomiting or diarrhea, your kidneys filter toxins out of the blood into urine, and your liver works hard to change the chemical nature of many toxins so they can be eliminated. If these systems are constantly having to work to detoxify your cells, however, they can get overwhelmed, and the toxins and waste can get backed up. Consuming contaminated water can cause nutrient deficiency, inflammation, swelling, weight gain, and immune system depletion.

When physical or chemical contaminants pollute a water source, the water becomes a potential risk for human health and can even transmit several dangerous diseases. Here are some common contaminants found in water:

+ **Microorganisms:** Bacteria, viruses, and protozoa can carry water-borne diseases such as cholera, typhoid fever, and gastroenteritis.
+ **Chemical pollutants:** Industrial activities, agricultural runoff, and improper disposal of chemicals can introduce pollutants like heavy metals (e.g., lead, mercury), pesticides, fertilizers, and pharmaceuticals into bodies of water.
+ **Organic matter:** Organic pollutants and contaminants like oil, grease, and organic solvents from urban runoff, industrial discharges, and sewage.

+ **Hormones and pharmaceuticals:** Residues of hormones, antibiotics, and other pharmaceuticals from human and animal waste can enter water sources through sewage and agricultural runoff.
+ **Household chemicals:** Improper disposal of household chemicals such as cleaning agents, paints, and batteries can lead to the contamination of groundwater and surface water sources.

These water contaminants can affect your health in many serious and often underrecognized ways.

The Effects of Contamination

Flint, Michigan, recently gained notoriety as the epicenter of a water access and public health crisis. Flint, home to General Motors (GM), had historically been a thriving hub for the automotive industry. Through the economic decline of the late twentieth century, the city, its population, and industries were hit hard.

To save costs, the city switched its water source from the Detroit Water and Sewerage Department to the Flint River in 2014. However, the city water department did not treat the Flint River water with an anticorrosive, and the water started leaching lead from the old pipes that supplied water to the city. The residents started complaining soon after the switch, but the government downplayed their concerns, insisting the water was safe to consume. The true severity of the problem came to light when multiple studies showed elevated levels of lead in the water.

Lead wreaks havoc in people's bodies by disturbing crucial cellular functions including enzyme activity for digestion, cell signaling, cell membrane security to keep things in and out, protection from oxidation reactions in cells, and even proper DNA copying. Ingested lead turns the inner workings of people's cells into a chaotic mess. These serious effects made Flint's water contamination a major crisis, especially for young people whose bodies were still developing.

Water Quality Today

Like the people of Flint, your body needs clean, unpolluted water to both stay well and prevent illness. Because water travels rapidly throughout your body, the effects of ingesting contaminated water ripple through every system, leading to immediate as well as delayed effects on your wellness. You could experience digestive illnesses, problems with your liver and kidneys, nervous system or reproductive effects, and chronic diseases such as cancer. A survey conducted by the Environmental Working Group showed that more than 50 percent of respondents see their tap water as unsafe, and 40 percent won't or can't drink it straight from the tap.[260]

A recent study by the U.S. Geological Survey found similar results: they estimated that at least 45 percent of the nation's tap water contains one or more types of per- and polyfluoroalkyl substances, or PFAS,[261] commonly found in cleaning products, nonstick cookware, shampoo, dental floss, and nail polish.[262] PFAS may increase cholesterol levels, decrease immune system responsiveness, negatively affect the liver, lead to lower birth weight in infants and preeclampsia in pregnant parents, and increase the risk of kidney or testicular cancer.[263] Making matters worse, most municipal systems are not designed to remove synthetic contaminants such as PFAS, glyphosate, and pharmaceuticals.[264]

Chlorine and Fluorine in Your Water

Clean water is essential for cellular health. It's important that the water you use for drinking, cooking, and hygiene is uncontaminated. Drinking water that comes from a treated municipal supply may be free of contaminants that will make you immediately unwell, but it still may have an unpleasant taste or smell and contain health-impacting chemicals such as chlorine or fluoride. Chlorine is commonly used in water treatment to disinfect and kill harmful microorganisms, but in drinking water, it can harm cells and negatively affect overall health. When chlorine reacts with other organic matter in the water, it can form molecules that damage cell membranes, proteins, and DNA, and can even cause direct damage to cells, leading to cell death in the respiratory tract and skin. It also forms by-products that have been linked to various health issues, including cancer and developmental problems.

Fluoride may be even more harmful to cells. As a dentist, I was trained to promote fluoride use to my patients. In dental school, I learned about its origins, and using it made sense. Dental and governmental agencies encouraged adding fluoride to water and dental products to decrease tooth decay. Fluoride does make teeth stronger, but like anything that you put in your body, it affects every cell, not just the tooth cells. Fluoride inhibits many cellular activities by binding to the enzyme receptor site on cells, effectively blocking the enzyme from doing its job.[265] Some potential side effects of fluoride on the body include:

+ Disruption of thyroid function, leading to hypothyroidism and goiters.[266]
+ Damage in the bone, brain, and kidneys.[267]
+ Hormone imbalances and birth defects.[268]

Most worrisome is the concern about the effect of fluoride on the neurodevelopment in children. In a startling study in the *Environmental Research* journal in 2023, researchers found higher fluoride levels directly correlated with lower IQ scores in children.[269] Is this risk worth the reward of stronger teeth? Absolutely not, especially because we have a fluoride alternative today that doesn't have these risky side effects: hydroxyapatite, the mineral complex that makes tooth enamel and bones. It is now being added to dental products in the place of fluoride, and studies find it to be equal to or better than fluoride at preventing tooth decay.[270] This is why I no longer recommend fluoride to patients or followers; there is too much unnecessary risk.

How to Get Clean Water

Thankfully, home water treatments can effectively clean your water of dozens of contaminants in a broad range of categories. The effects can be as minor as improving the taste of the water or as important as removing potential hazards to your wellness. It's important to remember that there is no one single treatment system that removes all contaminants, whether it's a pitcher with a filter or whole house filter system. A combination of treatment methods is necessary to get pure water. Let's take a look at some different types of water treatments:

Mechanical filters: Remove sand, dirt, rust, and waterborne parasites like giardia

Adsorption filters: Remove chemicals such as dyes, chlorine, pesticides, herbicides, and pharmaceuticals

Sequestration filters: Chemically isolate or trap contaminants

Ion exchange filters: Remove calcium and magnesium to "soften" hard water by exchanging the magnesium and calcium ions found in hard water with sodium or hydrogen ions

Reverse osmosis systems: Remove nearly all minerals, metals, chlorine, fluoride, other chemicals, and some bacteria and viruses

Boiling: Removes bacteria and viruses like giardia

Distillation: Removes minerals, metals, chemicals, bacteria, and viruses

Chemical purification (using chlorine or iodine): Kills bacteria, viruses, and some parasites

Ultraviolet (UV) light: Destroys bacteria, viruses, algae, mold, and some parasites

Water Purification Chart

The listed water purification methods can partially
indicated with (/) or fully remove the following impurities

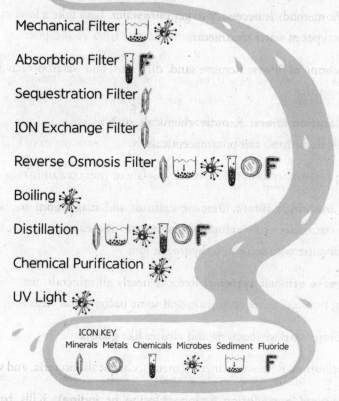

Each of these methods is used for different reasons. For example, distilled water is used if you need extreme purity, while filtered water is adequate for daily drinking. Each of these methods will leave your water purer and more able to carry what your cells need.

What kind of water is best for your wellness, energy, and cells? This question has led to an explosion of proposed "healthy water" options, including bottled water touting multiple health claims and a variety of expensive systems to modify water at home. To simplify all of these options, let's go back to what your cells need from water and how you can reproduce the positive benefits nature's water brings, right from your own home.

Drinking Well Practices

Supply

- ✦ At the very least, use mechanical and adsorption filters to remove microbes, chemicals, and some fluoride from your tap water.
- ✦ If using a reverse osmosis filter or distiller that removes all minerals, add electrolyte powder or drops to your water to return essential electrolytes back. These are necessary for proper nerve and muscle function as well as tooth and bone health.[271]
- ✦ Squeeze fresh citrus juice into your water to add vitamin C to support your immune system, help repair your tissues, improve your breakdown of food, and flush toxins out of the body.
- ✦ Take hot Epsom salt (magnesium sulfate) baths to gain magnesium that is crucial for cellular functions such as enzyme activity, energy production, and DNA synthesis.

Support

- ✦ Take cold plunges, which can reduce inflammation and muscle soreness and reduce swelling and tissue breakdown.[272]
- ✦ Switching between cold and warm water in the shower or bath boosts blood flow. Doing this for a few minutes a day or a few times a week can help your body recover faster, reduce soreness, and deliver more oxygen and nutrients to your cells.[273]
- ✦ Soak in a hot tub. The heat from hot tubs relaxes muscles and increases blood flow, which can aid in the delivery of oxygen and nutrients to cells, promoting healing and recovery.

Security

- ✦ Visit a sauna. Saunas can help eliminate toxins through sweat and improve circulation, which supports cellular health.

✦ Make sure to drink enough water. Simply getting enough water into your body is essential for cells to maintain their structural integrity, allowing for normal cellular processes including cell defenses.

Signals

✦ Add mineral-rich salt to a glass of water and shake or stir. This causes the minerals in the salt to separate, creating a flow of electrons that power up your cells.

✦ Ramp up the effects of grounding by putting your bare feet in a natural moving water source.

✦ Spend time near oceans, waterfalls, and other bodies of moving water. This can expose you to negative ions which give you and your cells more electrons. You can also purchase negative ion generators and salt lamps that release negative ions into the air.[274]

Simply put, the water element is very nourishing for cellular health and overall wellness. It encourages hydration and lubrication, supports cellular integrity and mobility, and literally helps every cell and every cellular function to work better. Water is a lifeline for your cells, delivering vital nutrients and efficiently removing waste. Forget the rigid rule of eight glasses a day; your body has a built-in reminder system called thirst. Listen to it. However, the quality of the water you consume is very important, as clean, contaminant-free water ensures your cells receive what they need without suffering damage. Incorporating water therapies such as cold plunges, hot tubs, and Epsom salts baths can further enhance your cellular health by boosting circulation, reducing inflammation, and promoting relaxation. Water is good for you and your cells and is a crucial part of your journey to wellness.

Chapter 9
Keyhole Concepts

- Water is crucial for health. It fuels your metabolism, gives your body its shape, and lubricates your movements. Water also carries nutrients and other "precious cargo" to every cell in your body.

- Water affects many of your senses and improves mental and overall health in a variety of ways.

- Water regulates many of your most important metabolic processes, including metabolism, digestion, circulation, and the making of cellular structures and components like proteins and DNA.

- If your cells need more water, your body has a very simple mechanism for letting you know. Put simply, you will get thirsty.

- Chlorine is often used to clean water for drinking. But when chlorine reacts with other organic matter in the water, it can form molecules that cause oxidative stress, damaging cell membranes, proteins, and DNA.

- Studies show hydroxyapatite is equal to or better than fluoride at preventing tooth decay. While fluoride does make teeth stronger, like anything that you put in our body, it affects every cell, not just the tooth cells. Ingesting it frequently can have negative side effects.

- To improve your tap water, use mechanical and adsorption filters to remove microbes and chemicals; if using a reverse osmosis filter or distiller that strips minerals, add electrolyte powder or drops to restore essential minerals; and add fresh citrus juice for vitamin C.

- It's important to remember that there is no one single treatment system that removes all contaminants.

- The water element is simply nourishing for cellular health and overall wellness. It encourages hydration and lubrication, supporting cellular integrity and mobility, and literally helps every cell and every cellular function to work better.

PART 3

Seasons of Wellness

Thomas Edison, the tireless tinkerer and celebrated inventor who jump-started the age of electric light, changed the world. But electric light bulbs haven't stayed the same since their invention; they have continued to evolve and improve. So has our understanding of how we stay well. The Cell Well model draws from all that has been used for centuries to help people stay well, combining traditional knowledge with ongoing modern advancements to continually evolve. The Seasons of Wellness will help you pull all the Cell Well principles and practices together and find your own next steps to take.

CHAPTER 10

Getting to Know the Seasons

In Part Two, you discovered how the Elements of Wellness can help you and your cells get more energy, or fire. As you read, you were probably wondering: How do I get started, and what will bring me benefit quickly? How can I jump-start my journey to being well?

Before you can answer those questions, let's consider a few other things:

+ What are the early warning signs that indicate things are not functioning well on a cellular level?
+ What is disease, and what happens to your cells to make them sick?

As we have learned, cells stay well if they have the supplies, support, security, and signals that they need. When your cells and body are out of balance in one of these areas, you know because you experience a symptom like pain, swelling, fever, fatigue, dizziness, or vomiting! Symptoms like these are the warning signs that your cells aren't well. If the imbalance isn't corrected, your cells honk their metaphorical horns, and do anything they can to get your attention. Stroke, heart disease, cancer, diabetes, Alzheimer's, autoimmune disease, gastrointestinal problems, etc., are all groups of warning signs your cells are sending. The imbalance at the cellular level caused the symptom, and the uncorrected symptoms led to what modern Western medicine calls disease. Your body is very resilient, however, and you probably have learned to adapt to many of the symptom messages your cells are sending you every day. This might be the headache you wake up with but drown in your morning cup of coffee, or the stiff joints and back that you explain away because you just had another birthday. Unfortunately, these adaptations and "explanations" mask when your cells are struggling.

Your Cells Get Tired Too: Meg's Story

Meg knew all about adapting. She was a beautiful singer and the host of a YouTube channel. Her voice was her livelihood, so when it started to fail, she desperately began looking for reasons why.

Meg originally lost her voice after fighting a nasty virus, but after she got better, her voice didn't return. Visits with doctors for her throat, her gut, her ears, and more led to inconclusive tests and pharmaceutical suggestions that caused more problems than they corrected. These were dead ends that ended in frustration and confusion. After we began working together, Meg and I realized the virus wasn't the root cause of her symptoms. That virus was the last straw. Her body had been bombarded with many insults: a hidden infection at the end of a tooth that had had a root canal, food sensitivities that aggravated her digestive system, sleepless nights with a new baby, and more. She had adapted to each of these things, but when the virus came along, her cells had adapted so much they just couldn't do it anymore.

Cells lose their ability to adapt to stressors over time as they accumulate damage to their DNA, proteins, and other cellular components. This cumulative damage can exhaust the cell's repair mechanisms, leaving the cell unable to cope with additional stress. This cellular exhaustion was the real problem that Meg was suffering from, and the symptoms she had been covering up for years couldn't be ignored any longer. Modern medicine may have treated the virus, but to return to wellness, Meg had to address the underlying problem. She had to give her body and cells what they had been lacking for some time.

As you have found out, if you can heal one cell, you can heal them all. Using the Elements of Wellness, you can correct imbalances by bringing your cells the crucial bioelectricity and raw materials necessary for proper function. But how can you put those Elements to work in your life? Let's use the Seasons of Wellness as your guide.

The Seasons of Wellness

The Seasons of Wellness system helps individuals self-evaluate their cellular needs and take steps toward personalized wellness. It combines knowledge from various traditional medicines—Ayurveda, traditional Chinese medicine, Western herbalism, and more—into an accessible framework. By identifying the Season you're in, along with the related Element and lifestyle adjustments, you can shift away from generic health advice to a personalized approach that honors the unique rhythms of your body.

Just as the seasons naturally cycle, so does your body, moving through periods of growth, rest, and renewal. Each Season represents a phase in your cellular needs, guiding you to adapt your wellness practices accordingly. Understanding and aligning with your current Season will empower you to support, sustain, and rejuvenate your cells, beginning a wellness journey that flows in harmony with your body's natural cycles. In the following chapters, you'll assess your current Season of Wellness and learn targeted practices to energize your cells.

Seasons of Wellness Guides

Each of the following guides can be used in many ways. Here are two primary approaches to utilizing the information.

1. **Staying Well:** Choose your Season. If you would like to stay well, start by reading the focus and description at the top of each Season guide. That will help you find the Season that is most appropriate for your individual needs right now. Then use that Season's

targeted Cell Well Recommendations to help your body and cells stay well.

2. **Addressing a Symptom:** Choose a system or organ. If you have symptoms you would like relief from, and need to support the corresponding system or organ, start by looking at each Season's primary and secondary organs until you find the one that most matches your symptoms. Then use the corresponding Cell Well Recommendations to help your body and cells return to wellness.

Spring: The Season of Creation, Change, and Hope

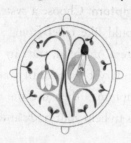

Spring is a time of rebirth, new growth, and expansion, mirroring the qualities of the plants Element. It is associated with renewal, flexibility, and the emergence of new possibilities.

When to Use This Guide

+ You are in a spring Season or your life and activities have spring characteristics.

Element: Plants

Focus: Healing, regeneration, connection, purpose.
Primary Organs: Liver, gallbladder. **Secondary Organs:** Tendons, eyes.

+ **Liver:** Nearly all the cleansing, processing, and movement of nutrients in your body happens in your liver.
+ **Gallbladder:** This organ stores and releases bile, which helps your body digest fats and supports the liver in eliminating fat-soluble toxins.

How You Feel in Spring

In Balance: Energetic, optimistic, creative, flexible, adaptable, decisive, emotionally balanced, self-aware, rejuvenated.

Out of Balance: Restless, irritable, frustrated, moody or temperamental, emotionally stuck.

Symptoms in Spring

In Balance

- Regular bowel movements
- No digestive discomfort
- Stable weight
- Clear vision
- Normal brown stool color
- Clear skin
- Balanced energy
- Vigor and vitality in daily life

Out of Balance

- Fatigue
- Poor appetite
- Bloating and gas
- Indigestion
- Nausea
- Eczema
- Unexplained weight gain
- Difficulty concentrating
- Anxiety or depression
- Blurry vision
- Muscle tension
- Cramps
- Lack of energy
- Uncomfortable fullness after meals
- Discomfort or pain under the right ribs
- Acne
- Itchy skin
- Yellowing of the skin and eyes
- Irritability
- Dry eyes
- Tension headaches
- Irregular menstrual cycles
- Infertility
- Mood swings

Spring Cell Well Recommendations

SUPPLY

Liver, Eyes, Tendons

✦ Eat greens that supply vitamins A, C, and K1 as well as folate and minerals including calcium, iron, and magnesium, which support liver function, vision, and tendon health.

1. Drink sixteen ounces of Cell Well Green Smoothie (page 293) for breakfast.
2. Try Oven-Roasted Broccoli (page 296) as a side for dinner.

✦ Incorporate sour flavors like citrus juices, vinegar, green apples, kimchi, and sauerkraut into your diet because they can stimulate liver function.

1. In the morning, drink sixteen ounces of water with the juice of one lemon.
2. Eat one green apple, sliced, every afternoon as a snack.

Gallbladder

✦ Reduce your consumption of fatty and fried foods, processed meats, soft drinks, and processed foods. Increase hydration by drinking more water.

1. Replace processed snack foods with apples, oranges, and carrots with hummus.
2. Drink water mixed with electrolyte powder in place of soft drinks.

✦ Add beets, carrots, dandelion greens, garlic, and onions to your meals.

1. Try Lemonade Beet Salad (page 298) as a side dish for dinner.

SUPPORT

Liver, Gallbladder, Tendons

✦ Include stretching, walking, yoga, or tai chi.

1. Take a thirty-minute walk three times a week.
2. Practice the Cell Well Spring yoga poses for fifteen minutes three times a week. Find poses at www.resources.livingwell book.com.

✦ Sleep is critical during the period from 11 PM to 3 AM, the gallbladder's and liver's peak active hours (page 274). Make sure to go to sleep by 11 PM.

✦ Use herbs to support and sustain the liver and gallbladder. Milk thistle, burdock, dandelion root, turmeric, and ginger all support healthy liver function. Drink eight ounces of Well Liver Tea (page 295) twice a day for five days.

SECURE

Liver, Gallbladder:

✦ Limit exposure to harmful chemicals in cleaning products, beauty products, and processed foods to reduce the liver's and gallbladder's detoxification burden.

1. Replace cleaning products with Well Home cleaning products (page 327).
2. Keep a spider plant in your home to help clean the air.

Eyes

✦ Natural light can help regulate your body's internal clock, improving eye health, sleep, and overall energy levels.

1. Open the window and spend some time outside or near a window every day.
2. When using a digital device, pause every twenty minutes to look at something twenty feet away for at least twenty seconds to reduce eye strain.

SIGNAL

Liver, Gallbladder, Eyes, Tendons

✦ To increase cell signaling, incorporate foods rich in omega-3 fatty acids, such as fatty fish (salmon, mackerel), flaxseeds, chia seeds, and walnuts. Drink the Chia Lime Refresher (page 295) as an afternoon pick-me-up twice a week.

✦ Increase magnesium intake. Magnesium is involved in hundreds of biochemical reactions in your body, including in cellular signaling pathways. Once a week, take a detox bath with magnesium-rich Epsom salts. Instructions can be found here (page 332).

✦ Try out acupressure. Apply pressure to points associated with the liver and gallbladder. Use Liver 3 and Gallbladder 34 once a day in the evening (page 338).

Summer: The Season of Movement and Growth

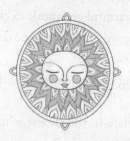

Together, summer and fire increase metabolic activity in every cell, provide internal heat, help your body digest food and process thoughts, and facilitate movement of nutrients through the heart and blood vessels.

When to Use This Guide

✦ You are in a summer Season or your life and activities have summer characteristics.

Element: Fire

Focus: Heat, transformation, energy, vitality.
Primary Organs: Heart, small intestine. **Secondary Organs:** Tongue, sweat glands.

✦ **Heart:** Summer and the fire Element govern both the physical and emotional heart as well as the health of your blood and blood vessels.
✦ **Small Intestine:** Fire and summer are connected not only to the digestion of food but also to your metabolism, the process that transforms food into energy.

How You Feel in Summer

In Balance: Energetic, passionate, social, adventurous, creative, playful, expressive, enthusiastic, optimistic, joyful, compassionate, empathetic, happy, calm, emotionally stable, peaceful.

Out of Balance: Emotionally unstable, anxious, restless, agitated, excessively excited, moody or temperamental, sensitive, impulsive, unusually reactive.

Symptoms in Summer

In Balance

- Normal blood pressure (around 120/80 mmHg)
- Regular heartbeat (between 60–100 beats per minute at rest)
- No chest pain
- Able to tolerate exercise
- No swelling
- Healthy weight
- Warm hands and feet
- No numbness
- Good endurance
- Restful sleep

Out of Balance

- Irregular heartbeat
- Chest pain
- High blood pressure (chronically higher than 130/85 mmHg)
- Intolerance of heat
- Profuse sweating
- Flushed
- Insomnia
- Difficulty falling asleep or staying asleep
- Overactive mind
- Excessive talking
- Speech disorders (stuttering)
- Rashes
- Eczema
- Hives
- Acne flare-ups
- Indigestion
- Acid reflux
- Diarrhea
- Excessive thirst
- Dry and red eyes
- Sensitivity to light
- Low sexual desire, arousal, or performance

Summer Cell Well Recommendations

SUPPLY

Heart, Small Intestine

✦ In summer, include cooling and hydrating foods in your diet to balance the heat of the fire Element.

1. Keep cut-up cucumbers and watermelon in the fridge to eat as a snack.
2. Make a Melon Refresher (page 307) with any melon of your choice.

✦ Avoid spicy, hot food and stimulants such as energy drinks and caffeine for at least a month.

✦ Bitter flavors can help counteract the heat and support heart and small intestine health. Make a salad with fresh arugula and drizzle olive oil and vinegar over the top.

✦ Drink plenty of water and other non-caffeinated beverages to stay hydrated.

1. In the summer, drink herbal teas at or slightly below room temperature. This keeps you from adding extra heat to your body and promotes a cooling effect. Try tea made from chrysanthemum, mint, honeysuckle, or hibiscus.
2. Do not drink ice-cold drinks, as they can shock the digestive system and impair your body's ability to break down and process food effectively, leading to digestive issues.

✦ Incorporate antioxidants into your meals to protect cells from oxidative stress caused by heat and increased activity. Berries, cherries, peaches, nectarines, tomatoes, and bell peppers are all great options. Try Tomato Cucumber Bruschetta for dinner tonight!

SUPPORT

Heart, Small Intestine, Sweat Glands

✦ Focus on less intense, cooling exercises like yoga, tai chi, or walking.

1. Take a walk in the early morning or late evening three times a week. Avoid high-intensity activities during peak heat hours (10 AM to 4 PM).

2. Spend fifteen minutes three times a week on the Cell Well Summer/Fire yoga poses that can be found at www.resources .livingwellbook.com

+ Summer is a good time to connect with others. Engage in social activities that foster joy and happiness at least once a week, as these are vital for nourishing the heart.

+ Getting enough sleep is crucial for health. Try to wake up earlier and go to bed later to align with the sun's pattern. Create a sleep schedule and stick to it.

+ Cooling herbs can be used in a tea to hydrate and support. Make a cup of chrysanthemum, hibiscus, rose, or hawthorn berry tea to cool down at midday.

SECURE

Heart, Small Intestine

+ While some spicy foods can promote circulation and open the pores to release sweat (thus cooling the body), excessive consumption can overheat the body. Limit spicy foods for one month to cool and balance the body.

+ Work to maintain a comfortable body temperature. This is particularly balancing for the fire Element.

1. Wear light, breathable clothing and take cool showers or baths.

2. Use fans or air conditioning and sleep with cool, breathable bedding to help regulate nighttime temperatures.

+ Coenzyme Q10 (CoQ10) can be beneficial for heart health and energy production at the cellular level. Take a CoQ10 supplement, if advised by your medicine practitioner.

SIGNAL

Heart, Small Intestine, Sweat Glands

✦ Stay out of the direct sun and wear loose, light-colored, and breathable clothing.

✦ Take cold plunges or cold showers. Cold exposure can activate brown adipose tissue, a type of fat that burns calories. Immerse yourself in cold water or take a cold shower for 1–2 minutes. Gradually increase the duration as you become more accustomed to the cold.

✦ Try acupressure. Apply pressure to the heart and small intestine points. Use the Heart 7 and 9 and Pericardium 7 and 9 points (page 340) and Small Intestine 3 and 8 points. Do this once a day in the evening.

✦ Maintaining a balance of electrolytes is crucial for cellular signaling, especially in the heart and small intestine. It's especially important in the hot summer to replenish what is lost from the sweat glands. Drink naturally electrolyte-rich beverages like coconut water, or make your own electrolyte water by adding a pinch of salt and a squeeze of lemon to your glass!

✦ Electromagnetic frequencies (EMF) disrupt cellular signaling and increase the incidence of disease.

1. Take device breaks and use EMF-blocking devices and shields when using electronic devices.

2. Turn off your Wi-Fi when it is not in use.

Harvest: The Season of Gathering, Reaping, and Plenty

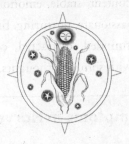

Harvest is a time for slowing down and gathering in. It's a time to stop and recognize where we get all that nourishes and sustains us, and to appreciate the abundance that the earth provides.

When to Use This Guide

+ You are in a harvest Season or your life and activities have harvest characteristics.

Element: Earth

Focus: Stability, nourishment, grounding.
Primary Organs: Spleen, stomach. **Secondary Organs:** Mouth, muscles, lymphatic system.

+ **Spleen:** The spleen filters your blood, removing old or damaged red blood cells, as well as bacteria and viruses. It also stores oxygen-carrying red blood cells, platelets that help with clotting, and white blood cells that are key defenders of your cells and body.
+ **Stomach:** The stomach plays a crucial role in the digestive process by storing, mixing, and breaking down food. It also provides a protective barrier against pathogens like bacteria, viruses, and parasites.

How You Feel in Harvest

In Balance: Grounded, content, stable, emotionally and physically nourished and balanced, compassionate, nurturing, full of abundance, peaceful.
Out of Balance: Absentminded, distracted, confused, forgetful, unfocused, worried, anxious, with spinning thoughts.

Symptoms in Harvest

In Balance

- Adequate stomach acid production
- Chewing is easy
- Regular bowel movements
- Healthy intestinal lining
- Steady energy levels
- No pain or discomfort after eating

Out of Balance

- Bloating and gas
- Acid reflux
- Discomfort from indigestion
- Heaviness, particularly after eating
- Lethargy
- Muscle atrophy
- Weakness
- Swelling (particularly in the lower extremities)
- Heaviness in the limbs
- Weight gain
- Cravings for sweet or starchy foods
- Frequent infections
- Difficulty losing weight (particularly around the abdomen)
- Irregular menstrual cycles
- Pale complexion
- Symptoms of premenstrual syndrome (PMS)
- Fertility issues
- Joint pain or stiffness (particularly in the knees and lower back)

Harvest Cell Well Recommendations

SUPPLY

Stomach, Spleen, Lymphatic System, Muscles

✦ Eat a variety of colorful fruits and vegetables including leafy greens like spinach, kale, and Swiss chard as well as root vegetables like carrots, sweet potatoes, and beets for vitamins, minerals, and anti-oxidants. Use cooking methods that preserve the nutritional value of the food, such as steaming, roasting, or lightly sautéing it.

1. Follow the thirty-minute Well Bowl Formula (page 309) for a colorful meal in just a few minutes.
2. Make Oven-Roasted Root Vegetables (page 311) for a mineral-rich meal.

✦ Incorporate beans, lentils, and chickpeas into your meals for plant-based protein, fiber, and various other nutrients. Try Six-Can Chili (page 298) for a quick-to-the-table meal full of healthy legumes.

✦ Include sources of healthy fats such as avocados, nuts, seeds, and olive oil in your diet to support cell structure and function. Make a batch of Cell Well Granola (page 312) and top it with almond milk for a tasty, healthy breakfast.

✦ Use herbs and spices like turmeric, ginger, garlic, and cinnamon, which not only add flavor but also provide health benefits. Try Chicken Tikka Masala (page 313) for a restaurant-worthy home-cooked dinner.

✦ Incorporate fermented foods like sauerkraut, kimchi, kefir, and yogurt into your diet. These foods contain probiotics that support stomach health and overall immune function. Use sauerkraut or yogurt as a topper on roasted potatoes for a double dose of stomach- and spleen-healthy foods.

✦ Minimize intake of processed foods, sugary snacks, and beverages high in added sugars. Challenge yourself to three days without added sugars and see how you feel.

SUPPORT

Stomach, Spleen, Muscles, Mouth

+ Spend time outdoors walking barefoot on grass, sand, or soil to practice grounding.
  1. Intentionally touch the earth for at least ten minutes per day. Walk, sit, or play on it while barefoot.
  2. Acquire a grounding pad, sheets, or shoes to bring yourself into contact with the earth more often.
+ Practice mindful eating, which allows for better digestion and absorption of nutrients from food. Once a day, slow down and pay attention to your eating. Savor each bite, chew food thoroughly, and pay attention to hunger and fullness cues.
+ Practice stress management techniques such as meditation, deep breathing exercises, yoga, or spending time in nature. Chronic stress can negatively impact cellular health and weaken the immune system Practice Cell Well Harvest/Earth yoga poses three times a week (page 336). Find the poses at www.resources.livingwellbook.com

Lymphatic System

+ Dry brush your skin regularly to stimulate lymphatic flow and remove dead skin cells. Use a natural bristle brush and use gentle strokes, always moving towards the heart. Do twice a week before showering (page 332).
+ Alternate between hot and cold water in the shower to improve circulation and support lymphatic drainage. Start with hot water for a few minutes, then switch to cold water for thirty seconds to one minute. Repeat the process several times. Try during every shower for a week.
+ Stimulate lymphatic flow to reduce swelling or congestion.
  1. Schedule regular lymphatic drainage massages with a qualified therapist.
  2. Avoid wearing tight clothing, especially around areas where lymph nodes are concentrated (e.g., groin, armpits), as it can restrict lymphatic flow.

SECURE

Stomach, Spleen, Lymphatic System, Muscles, Mouth

✦ Consider growing your own fruits, vegetables, and herbs, either in a backyard garden or in pots on a balcony or windowsill, or visit a local farm stand or farmer's market.

✦ Opt for organic and non-genetically modified organism (non-GMO) foods whenever possible to minimize exposure to pesticides, herbicides, and other harmful chemicals that can disrupt cellular function and overall health. Prioritize organic for foods that have been found to have high levels of contamination using the EWG's latest Clean Fifteen list, found at www.ewg.org.

✦ Ensure that your drinking water is clean and free from contaminants by using a high-quality water filtration system. Use the information you learned earlier about water filters in chapter 9 to select a filtration method and incorporate it into your daily hydration routine.

✦ Limit exposure to or consider using EMF protection devices for electromagnetic radiation from electronic devices such as cell phones, laptops, and Wi-Fi routers.

SIGNAL

Stomach, Spleen, Lymphatic System, Muscles, Mouth

✦ Include foods high in polyphenols, such as green tea, cocoa, dark chocolate, and spices like turmeric and cinnamon, along with adaptogenic herbs like ashwagandha, rhodiola, and ginseng into your routine. Start off your day with Dr. Michelle's Adaptogenic Golden Milk (page 314) instead of coffee for a week.

✦ Eat regular meals that include complex carbohydrates, healthy fats, and protein to help stabilize blood sugar levels. Fluctuations in blood sugar can affect cellular signaling pathways related to metabolism and energy production.

✦ Prioritize quality sleep to support cellular repair and optimize signaling processes. Aim for seven to nine hours of uninterrupted sleep each night and establish a relaxing bedtime routine.

✦ Acupuncture: Apply pressure to the Spleen 6 and 9 and Stomach 36 points (page 340). Do this once a day in the evening.

Fall: The Season of Release, Clearing, and Reflection

Fall is a time for letting go of what is unnecessary or what has served its purpose, both physically and emotionally. It's a period for clearing out, providing an opportunity to release old patterns or habits and make space for new growth.

When to Use This Guide

+ You are in a fall Season or your life and activities have fall characteristics.

Element: Air

Focus: Transition, reflection, balance.
Primary Organs: Lungs, large intestine. **Secondary Organs:** Skin, hair, nose, immune system.

+ **Lungs:** Fall is also a time to take in the pure and new with every breath you take. The lungs bring air and oxygen, the element that helps every cell make energy, into your body and your cells.
+ **Large Intestines (Colon):** The large intestines have the function of eliminating what is unnecessary or toxic from your body. They filter and process necessary nutrients, then expel the rest.

How You Feel in Fall

+ **In Balance:** Mentally clear, good at problem-solving and decision-making, emotionally resilient, efficient, disciplined, able to maintain healthy routines and boundaries, appreciative of beauty, spiritual, connected to heritage, drawn to growth, open to emotional release, creative, expressive.

+ **Out of Balance:** Grieving, sad, melancholic, plagued by perfectionism, unable to adapt to change.

Symptoms in Fall

In Balance

- "Breathing easy"
- No respiratory infections
- Regular bowel movements
- Physically strong, with good endurance

Out of Balance

- Coughing and wheezing
- Asthma attacks
- Shortness of breath
- Hay fever
- Colds, flu, and respiratory infections
- Dry skin
- Worsening allergy symptoms
- Psoriasis
- Eczema
- Bloating
- Acne
- Discomfort in your joints (particularly shoulders, arms, or hands)
- Constipation or diarrhea
- Low energy levels

Fall Cell Well Recommendations

SUPPLY

Lung, Nose, Immune System, Skin, Hair

+ Deep breathing exercises help strengthen and fully utilize the lungs and increase oxygen supply to the bloodstream.

    1. Practice deep breathing techniques every day in the morning to improve lung capacity and oxygen uptake. Follow the Well Lung Breathing Exercises (page 334).

    2. Spend time outdoors in natural environments where air quality is good and oxygen levels are higher.

+ Drink plenty of water throughout the day to maintain optimal hydration levels. Adequate hydration supports blood circulation, which is essential for transporting oxygen to cells. While there is no rule for the number of cups of water to drink per day, you need to pay attention to your hydration. Have water on hand to drink when you're thirsty and add electrolytes to increase the minerals the water brings to your cells.

+ Consume foods rich in oxygen-promoting nutrients such as iron, magnesium, and chlorophyll. These foods include leafy greens, cruciferous vegetables, berries, nuts, seeds, and omega-3 fatty acids found in fish.

    1. Make a Cellular Oxygen Smoothie in the morning for breakfast (page 317).

    2. Make Everyone's Favorite Spinach Salad for dinner and keep your cells and family happy (page 318).

+ Consider taking herbal supplements help improve circulation, enhance oxygen utilization, and support overall cellular health. Ginseng, ginkgo biloba, astragalus, and green tea extract are all supplements that can improve your circulation and oxygen usage.

Immune System

✦ Consume foods rich in immune-boosting nutrients like vitamin C, vitamin D, zinc, and selenium, as well as probiotics. Focus on citrus fruits, ginger, garlic, yogurt, and spinach.

1. Make Cold-Busting Ginger-ade (page 318) whenever you feel a sore throat coming on.
2. Take an elderberry supplement every day during season changes to ward off illness.

Large Intestine

✦ Fiber is crucial for promoting regular bowel movements and keeping the large intestine healthy. Aim to include a variety of high-fiber foods in your diet, such as oats, brown rice, quinoa, lentils, chickpeas, apples, berries, broccoli, carrots, spinach, dates, and garlic bananas.

1. Eat an apple with two dates for an afternoon snack.
2. Make Creamy Cell Well Hummus for a side dish or snack (page 320).

SUPPORT

Lung, Immune System, Nose, Skin, Hair

✦ Engage in regular aerobic exercises such as walking, jogging, swimming, or cycling to improve cardiovascular health, increase lung capacity, and enhance oxygen delivery to cells.

1. Find an exercise partner that can encourage you to do aerobic exercise at least twice per week.
2. Incorporate movement into your daily routine. Even simple activities like taking the stairs instead of the elevator or going for short walks can help.

✦ Good posture allows for better lung expansion and oxygen intake.
  1. Practice sitting and standing with your shoulders back and spine aligned to optimize breathing.
  2. Try doing wall angels (see appendix 4 of this book) twice per week to strengthen back and shoulder muscles.
✦ Practice stress-reducing techniques to promote relaxation and digestive and immune health. Mindfulness meditation, deep breathing exercises, yoga, and tai chi can all provide these benefits. Find poses at www.resources.livingwellbook.com

SECURE

Lung, Immune System, Nose

✦ Improve indoor air quality by using air purifiers or indoor plants that help filter out pollutants and increase oxygen levels indoors. See Breathing Well Guide for air purifier recommendations (page 202).
  1. Bring an English ivy, peace lily, palm, snake plant, Boston fern, or spider plant into your home to clean the air.
  2. Minimize exposure to air pollutants such as cigarette smoke, vehicle emissions, and industrial pollutants by watching the air warnings where you live and staying inside when the quality is poor.
✦ Pay attention to your hygiene. Wash your hands regularly, avoid close contact with sick individuals, and cover your mouth and nose when coughing or sneezing.

Hair, Skin

✦ Use natural personal care products to reduce toxin exposure. Try recipes from the Well Body Products list at home (page 329).

SIGNAL

Lung, Immune System

✦ Ensure you get enough restful sleep each night to support cellular repair and regeneration.

1. Make sure you are sleeping between 3 AM and 5 AM for healthy lung recovery.

✦ Incorporate healthy fats into your diet, such as omega-3 fatty acids found in fatty fish, flaxseeds, chia seeds, and walnuts. Eat foods rich in phospholipids, such as eggs, soybeans, sunflower seeds, and peanuts.

1. Try Miso Glazed Salmon for a delicious cell-healthy dinner (page 321).

2. Make Cell Well No-Bake Cookies and keep them in the fridge to grab and go (page 322).

✦ Use acupressure. Apply pressure to the lung and large intestine points. Use Lung 7 and Large Intestine 4 points. (See Appendix 4 of this book.) Do this once a day in the evening.

Winter: The Season of Rest, Resilience, and Renewal

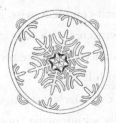

Winter offers opportunities for rest and reflection. It also offers the opportunity to gather with friends and family. Winter reminds people about the cyclical nature of life. No matter how long and cold winter may seem, spring is always on the way.

When to Use This Guide

+ You are in a winter Season or your life and activities have winter characteristics.

Element: Water

Focus: Rest, regeneration, cleansing.
Primary Organs: Kidneys, bladder. **Secondary Organs:** Ears, bones, teeth, reproductive organs.

+ **Kidneys:** Your kidneys regulate water metabolism and stabilize the heart and blood pressure. They revitalize your body by separating and circulating clean water and eliminating contaminated water.
+ **Bladder:** Your bladder is the reservoir in your body where water collects. Every few seconds, urine is passed from the kidneys to the bladder, where it is stored until it is eliminated through urination. When the bladder is not functioning optimally, your entire system is in danger of backing up with toxic wastes.

How You Feel in Winter

+ **In Balance:** Vital, strong, enduring, courageous, able to overcome fear and adversity, self-confident, wise, insightful, able to learn from past experience, connected with your inner self, flexible, adaptable, confident in your ability to navigate life's changes, resilient, spiritually connected, healthily aging.

+ **Out of Balance:** Excessively fearful, anxious, insecure, tending towards emotionally withdrawing, isolated, detached from others and the world.

Symptoms of Winter

In Balance

- Strong bones and teeth
- Regular menstruation
- Healthy sperm quality and libido
- Easy to eliminate urinary waste
- Agile
- Smooth movement in your joints, muscles, and tissues
- Deep, restorative sleep patterns
- Rejuvenated body and mind

Out of Balance

- Chronically tired
- Lacking energy
- Sense of being depleted
- Osteoporosis
- Joint pain
- Stiffness (particularly in the lower back, knees, ankles)
- Struggle with infertility
- Low libido
- Irregular menstruation
- Erectile dysfunction
- Frequent urination
- Urinary urgency
- Wake up at night to urinate
- Chronic or acute lower back pain
- Weakness
- Discomfort
- Tinnitus
- Hearing loss
- Ear infections
- Hair loss or premature graying
- Frequent infections (urinary tract or respiratory)
- Weak or brittle teeth

Winter Cell Well Recommendations

SUPPLY

Kidney, Bladder, Reproductive Organs

+ Drink plenty of water throughout the day to support kidney function and maintain hydration levels in the bladder. Always have a water bottle with you filled with clean, filtered water.

    1. Reduce consumption of caffeine, alcohol, and salt, as they can dehydrate the body and place additional strain on the kidneys and bladder. Substitute a natural energy stimulant like mushroom coffee for energy.

    2. Citrus fruits like oranges, lemons, and grapefruits are rich in vitamin C, which can help acidify urine and prevent the formation of kidney stones. Drink fresh citrus juice to prevent and eliminate kidney stones.

+ Berries such as blackberries, blueberries, strawberries, and raspberries may help protect against urinary tract infections and support kidney health. Treat your body and your cells with No-Bake Fruit Crumble (page 323).

+ Eat foods that regulate bowel movements and help increase urine production and cleaning. Juice half a bunch of celery first thing in the morning and drink before eating anything else.

    1. Try Healthy Kidney Black Bean Soup to help with kidney function (page 324).

    2. Make homemade Cell Well Miso soup (page 325).

Bones, Teeth

+ Ensure adequate intake of vitamin D3 through sunlight exposure and/or supplementation, as it is essential for calcium absorption and tooth and bone health.

    1. Eat butter made from grass-fed cows for a good source of vitamin D3 and K2 or take 5,000 IU of vitamin D3 and 1,000 mcg of vitamin K2 as supplements when needed for dental health.

2. Use a hydroxyapatite-containing tooth powder for cleaning teeth (see www.livingwellwithdrmichelle.com).

3. Limit sugary and acidic foods and beverages, as they can contribute to tooth decay and weaken bone density.

4. Substitute Chia Lime Refresher (page 295) for a sugary soft drink.

SUPPORT

Kidney, Bladder, Reproductive Organs

✦ Consider herbal remedies such as dandelion root, parsley, and nettle leaf, which have diuretic properties that can support kidney health and urinary tract function. Make a cup of dandelion or nettle tea and drink it warm every morning.

✦ Engage in regular physical activity to support circulation, hormone balance, and overall well-being.

1. Aim for a mix of cardiovascular exercise, strength training, and flexibility exercises.

2. Find time for thirty minutes of moderate-intensity exercise at least four days per week. Use the Well Week Exercise Guide if you need a path (page 338).

✦ Empty your bladder regularly to prevent urinary stasis and reduce the risk of urinary tract infections. Focus on avoiding holding your urine for prolonged periods.

1. Use herbal teas and supplements such as cranberry extract or dandelion root, which may support urinary tract health and kidney function.

2. Try drinking eight ounces of cranberry juice (not cranberry juice cocktail) per day to prevent or help with a urinary tract infection. Dilute with water if the flavor is too strong.

✦ Practice stress-reduction techniques such as meditation, yoga, deep breathing exercises, or mindfulness to help manage stress levels and support urinary and reproductive health. Practice Cell Well Winter/Water yoga poses. Find at www.resources.livingwellbook.com.

Ears

+ Use herbal ear drops containing ingredients like mullein oil, garlic oil, or tea tree oil to soothe and support ear health. If approved by a health-care professional, use mullein or garlic oil drops in each ear twice daily. (Please consult with a health-care professional before using any ear drops, especially if you have a history of ear problems.)

Teeth, Bones

+ Clean teeth daily with a hydroxyapatite-containing tooth product. Use twice per day and make sure to let the hydroxyapatite sit on the teeth for ten minutes before rinsing (see www.livingwellwith drmichelle.com).
+ Clean between the teeth with floss, a water flosser, or small flexible picks to protect teeth from decay.

SECURE

Teeth

+ Use coconut oil or another mild-flavored oil to "oil pull." This practice helps defend teeth from bacteria and balance the oral and gut microbiome. Put one tablespoon of oil in the mouth and swish in and out of the teeth for ten to fifteen minutes. Spit into a tissue and discard. Repeat daily for three days, then every third day as needed.

Ears

+ Protect your ears from extreme temperatures and injury.
  1. Avoid putting cotton swabs or other objects into the ear canal, as this can push wax deeper inside and increase the risk of injury or infection. Gently clean the outer ear with a damp cloth whenever you shower or bathe.
  2. Wear hats or earmuffs in cold weather and use earplugs while swimming or bathing to prevent infections.

Kidney, Bladder, Reproductive Organs

✦ Wear appropriate clothing to keep warm and protect these organs from cold temperatures.

✦ Consider using a heating pad or warm compress to provide comfort and promote blood flow to these organs during colder months.

SIGNAL

Reproductive Organs

✦ Support hormonal balance through herbs such as chasteberry (also known as vitex), maca root, and evening primrose oil. Add two teaspoons of maca root and one teaspoon of primrose oil to your morning smoothie.

✦ Take action to avoid endocrine-disrupting chemicals including BPAs, phthalates, parabens, and glyphosate. Find personal care products that don't contain phthalates or parabens.

1. Use a glass water bottle instead of a plastic one.
2. Buy organic as much as possible when eating the outside of a food to avoid glyphosate exposure.

Kidney, Bladder

✦ Empty your bladder regularly to help maintain healthy signaling in the urinary tract. When the bladder is allowed to empty frequently, the nerves that signal fullness and control urination stay active and responsive, supporting better urinary health and reducing the risk of infections and urinary retention issues.

✦ Use acupressure. Apply pressure to the kidney and bladder points, Kidney 1 and Spleen 6 and 9 (see appendix 4 of this book). Do this once a day in the evening.

Seasons of Wellness Guides Recap

Now that we've introduced the Seasons of Wellness guides, we can move into the Seasons Assessment, where you can get started on building your personalized path to wellness. Using where you are in the Seasons and these guides, you can now begin to supply, support, secure, and signal your cells through the Cell Well model.

All the resources listed in the Seasons guides are in the appendices in the back of this book. Also make sure to visit www.resources.livingwellbook .com for updated and additional recommendations as well as downloadable PDFs of the guides and included resources.

Congratulations—you are on your way to personalized cell wellness!

CHAPTER 11

What's Your Season?

Which Season are you and your cells in right now? The Seasons of Wellness Assessment will help you find out, and it will give you your starting place for your personalized Cell Well practice.

The Assessment is simple. Focusing on your present symptoms, make an X next to every symptom your cells are expressing right now (some symptoms may appear more than once). After you've done that, tally the total number of Xs for each column and put the number into the Total box at the bottom of that column. Remember to use your present symptoms, not ones you had in the past and that have now cleared up. The Seasons of Wellness Assessment is about where you are now, not where you have been or where you want to be. There are no right or wrong or good or bad results.

Seasons of Wellness Assessment

Place a mark in the space next to every symptom you are experiencing right now.				
Column 1	Column 2	Column 3	Column 4	Column 5
Indigestion	Bloating	Discomfort after eating	Asthma	Hair and teeth problems
Irritable bowels	Gas	Diarrhea	Shortness of breath	Sexual dysfunction
Dull skin	Nausea	Bloating	Susceptibility to respiratory infections	Irregular menstruation
Slow recovery after injury	Heart palpitations/irregular heartbeat	Poor nutrient absorption	Weak immune system	Difficulty urinating
Jaw clenching	Poor circulation	Poor appetite	Nasal congestion	Achy lower back pain
Dizzy spells	Lack of joy/passion	Fatigue	Sore throat	Feelings of insecurity
Headaches	Depression	Lethargy	Dry skin	Fatigue
Muscle spasm	Emotional instability	Excessive Worry	Constipation	Excessive fear
Brittle nails	Mental fog	Overthinking	Difficulty letting go	Reproductive issues
Stubbornness	Lack of focus	Scattered thoughts	Attachment to grudges	Cognitive decline
Lack of motivation	Forgetfulness	Low self-esteem	Rigid beliefs	Cold hands/feet
Muscle stiffness	Heartburn	Cravings for sweets/starches	Perfectionism	Excessive urination
Poor circulation	Acid reflux	Muscle weakness	Excessive focus on details	Excessive dryness
Neck pain	Rapid heart rate	Weight gain	Allergies	Dehydration

Muscle tightness	High blood pressure	Fluid retention	Sinusitis	Infertility
Stiff joints	Excessive sweating	Feelings of overwhelm	Chronic bronchitis	Enlarged prostate
Difficulty setting/achieving goals	Heatstroke	Lack of focus	Detachment	Insomnia
Fatigue	Dehydration	Stubbornness	Aloofness	Early graying
Irritability	Hyperactivity	Poor memory	Lack of empathy	Waking frequently during the night
Blurred/red/dry/itchy eyes	Restlessness	Anxiety	Cough/colds	Waking up at night to urinate
Menstrual cycle imbalance	Insomnia	Disorganization	Lower back pain	Paranoia
Rigidity of the tendons	Anxiety	Sense of confusion	Sinus infection	Feeling of withdrawal
Overly judgmental feelings	Irritability	Dependent on others	Diarrhea	Excessive rest
Feelings of stagnation	Manic behavior	Mood swings	Chest congestion	Stiffness
Struggles with make decisions	Outburst of anger	Emotional sensitivity	Scattered thoughts	Mental exhaustion
Attachment to old habits	Agitated/chaotic	Difficulty concentrating	Energy fluctuations	Poor memory
Total:	Total:	Total:	Total:	Total:

Reading Your Results

Each of the columns of the Seasons of Wellness Assessment corresponds to one of the five Seasons and Elements. To avoid overwhelm, you are going to start with one Season/Element only.

1. Find the column that has the highest total number of marks. If your highest number of marks is in:
   + **Column 1:** You will start with Spring/Plants.
   + **Column 2:** You will start with Summer/Fire.
   + **Column 3:** You will start with Harvest/Earth.
   + **Column 4:** You will start with Fall/Air.
   + **Column 5:** You will start with Winter/Water.

   Once you've determined your Season/Element starting point, take a close look at that column.

2. Tally the number of marks in the upper, darker-shaded area. Then tally the number of marks in the lower, lighter-shaded area. If you see more marks in the:
   + lower, lighter-shaded section of the column, you have an excess of that Element.
   + upper, darker shaded section of the column, you have a deficiency of that Element.

* To get a fillable PDF or online interactive version of the Seasons of Wellness Assessment, visit www.resources.livingwellbook.com.

Using Your Results

The Seasons of Wellness Assessment is the key to your personalized path to wellness. Instead of lists, charts or three-day, thirty-day, or longer "plans" or "programs," the Cell Well model starts you on a path that's suited to your individual needs and that you can traverse at your own speed. You can also take any side paths you find that interest you along the way.

Seasons Snapshot

The Seasons Snapshot gives you a quick way to identify which season is most associated with the organ, symptom, or life situation you are experiencing. Take a look at the picture and find which season best represents your current state.

In the following pages, we'll demonstrate how to use this information through two examples. Then you can use the Snapshot (along with last chapter's in-depth Season guides) to apply the information to your own wellness situation.

Seasons Snapshot

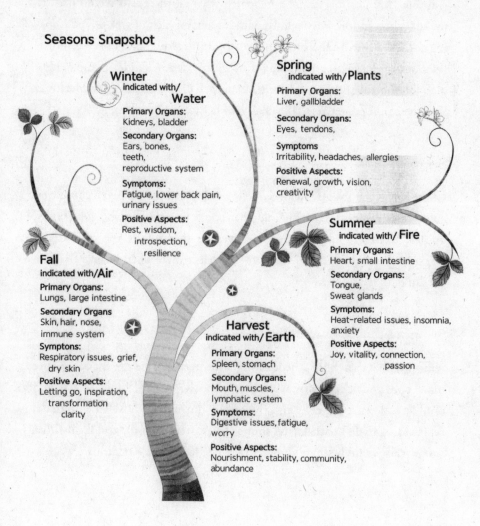

Winter
indicated with/ **Water**

Primary Organs:
Kidneys, bladder

Secondary Organs:
Ears, bones,
teeth,
reproductive system

Symptoms:
Fatigue, lower back pain,
urinary issues

Positive Aspects:
Rest, wisdom,
introspection,
resilience

Spring
indicated with/ **Plants**

Primary Organs:
Liver, gallbladder

Secondary Organs:
Eyes, tendons,

Symptoms:
Irritability, headaches, allergies

Positive Aspects:
Renewal, growth, vision,
creativity

Summer
indicated with/ **Fire**

Primary Organs:
Heart, small intestine

Secondary Organs:
Tongue,
Sweat glands

Symptoms:
Heat-related issues, insomnia,
anxiety

Positive Aspects:
Joy, vitality, connection,
passion

Fall
indicated with/ **Air**

Primary Organs:
Lungs, large intestine

Secondary Organs
Skin, hair, nose,
immune system

Symptons:
Respiratory issues, grief,
dry skin

Positive Aspects:
Letting go, inspiration,
transformation
clarity

Harvest
indicated with/ **Earth**

Primary Organs:
Spleen, stomach

Secondary Organs:
Mouth, muscles,
lymphatic system

Symptoms:
Digestive issues, fatigue,
worry

Positive Aspects:
Nourishment, stability, community,
abundance

Let's take a closer look at how this works in practice.

Proactively Improving Wellness: Claire's Busy Month

Claire knew she was facing a stressful month. It was May, jokingly called "May-cember" by other moms like her with school-aged kids.

The family calendar was packed with activities, gatherings, and ceremonies, and little time for rest in between. Knowing she and the kids would be running around a lot, Claire anticipated what all their cells would need to make it through the busy month without getting sick or run-down. Looking at the Seasons Snapshot, Claire realized this would be a busy "summer-like" Season for her family. Using the summer Season guide, Claire made a plan for boosting her family's wellness in each Cell Well category. She loved that she could proactively take charge of her family's wellness.

Supply

Claire knew that she and her kids' cells would need easy to digest foods that could provide energy quickly and that could be eaten on the go: **grapes, apples, oranges, cucumbers, and watermelon** all fit the bill. Claire stocked up on these light, vitamin- and electrolyte-filled snacks that are easy to grab in a hurry.

Support

Knowing that their busy schedule might mean they'd have to eat out, Claire made conscious choices to avoid heavy, greasy, or fried foods that would only slow down their cells and the family during this busy time. **Salads, restaurant-made broth-based soups (like tortilla soup), and fruit-filled smoothies** would be their go-tos if they needed a take-out meal.

Secure

Claire also planned ahead and chose supplements that would strengthen her family's immune systems to keep them well. The last thing they needed this month was to get sick! **Elderberry concentrate diluted in water**, a yummy preventive drink that helps build immune defenses, was exactly what Claire and her family needed.

Signal

Claire knew how tired she and her kids could get this time of year. **Electrolyte powder dissolved in water** was Claire's go-to when she noticed that she or the kids were dragging and needed more energy.

Remember, the first goal of the Cell Well model is to *stay* well by preserving and increasing wellness in every cell. Claire's proactive approach helped her family do just that. However, it's not always possible to head off cell symptoms. The most important thing to remember is that when your cells send you signals that they aren't well in the form of symptoms, your first response should not be to cover up those symptoms, but to use the Cell Well model to help your cells *return* to wellness.

Returning to Wellness by Listening to Symptoms: Jae's Sore Ear

Jae went to a concert, and as he walked back to his car in the chilly air, his left ear started to ache. Blaming it on the loud music and the cool spring weather, Jae didn't worry about it until the next morning, when swallowing hurt. He realized he must be "getting sick."

Rather than resigning himself to a miserable week, letting whatever he had "caught" run its course, Jae was determined to give his cells what they needed to quickly get past what was ailing them. Using the Seasons

Snapshot, Jae realized he was dealing with a Winter/Water problem. By choosing and implementing one recommendation from each category from the winter Season guide, he cleared up his symptoms in three days—quickly enough to go on a hike with friends that weekend!

Supply

Winter foods are dark blue and black. **Blueberries, blackberries, and black bean soup** filled Jae's shopping cart and meals. They support winter related organs, ears, and kidneys.

Support

Jae avoided excessive salt, sugar, and dairy, including **salty pretzels, tortilla chips, and dairy ice cream, to alleviate stress on his system.**

Secure

Jae started using garlic oil, a potent antibacterial and antiviral treatment, in his ear four times a day.

Signal

Electrolytes in water were the best of both worlds for Jae—electrons for signals and energy and water to help his systems, especially his kidneys. He drank two bottles of electrolyte-filled water each day.

CHAPTER 12

Wellness Applied: How to Live Well

Everyone deserves to be well. Yet not all of us have the expertise to decipher the complexities of modern or traditional medicine. That's exactly why this chapter is full of practical, easy-to-understand next steps, designed to support your journey toward wellness using the Cell Well model. Whether you're taking small steps or giant leaps, you'll find the perfect starting point in the next chapters and in the appendices. They contain everything you'll need for your journey to help your cells get well and stay well.

Seasons of the Day

The Seasons can be used to help you live well every single day. Each part of the day aligns with a natural Element, and understanding this can help you optimize your wellness choices from sunrise to sunset.

1. **Spring:** Begin your day by incorporating plant foods into your morning meal. These foods act as natural cleansers, preparing your body for the day's activities by flushing out toxins.

2. **Summer:** In midday, your body's energy shifts into the high gear of summer. Your digestive fire peaks, making it the ideal time to eat a nutrient-dense lunch to process and power the rest of your day.

3. **Harvest:** In the afternoon, you transition into the nourishing time of harvest. Your body is now distributing the vital nutrients you consumed earlier to the cells that need them most, fueling your ongoing activities and maintaining your energy balance.

4. **Fall:** The evening is a time for winding down as your body begins its nightly cleansing process, removing waste and slowing its rhythms in preparation for rest.

5. **Winter:** Finally, during the night your body enters a deep state of rest, repair, and rejuvenation, preparing you for the fresh start that awaits with the dawn.

When you harness the wisdom of the Seasons and Elements each day and let these ancient rhythms guide your dietary and lifestyle choices, you'll enhance your wellness in a way that's both natural and effective.

Seasons of the Day Guides

SEASONS OF THE DAY

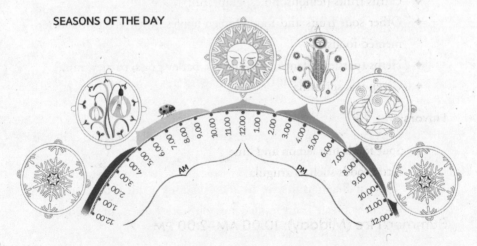

The following are guides for how to fuel and care for your cells and body during the cycle of the day.

Spring/Plants (Morning): 5:00 AM–10:00 AM

Mindfulness: Express gratitude and set intentions for your wellness. Consider journaling or writing down your goals for the day.

Activities: Gentle stretching exercises or a short walk to awaken your body and increase circulation.

Nutrition:

1. First thing, drink a glass of water with the juice of one lemon added. Wait thirty minutes before having breakfast.
2. Enjoy a nutritious breakfast of plant-based carbohydrates, proteins, and healthy fats. Oatmeal topped with nuts and fruit, a veggie omelet with avocado, or a smoothie made with leafy greens and fruit are good options.

Foods: Choose these foods in the morning:

+ Leafy greens (spinach, kale, lettuce, Swiss chard)
+ Sprouts (alfalfa, bean sprouts)
+ Green vegetables (asparagus, broccoli, green beans, artichokes, green peas, celery)
+ Citrus fruits (lemons, limes, grapefruit)
+ Other sour fruits and foods (green apples, kiwi, vinegar, and fermented foods)
+ Herbs (parsley, cilantro, wheatgrass, barley grass, parsley, mint)
+ Green tea, spirulina

Flavors:

+ Sour foods like lemon and lime
+ Bitter foods such as arugula

Summer/Fire (Midday): 10:00 AM–2:00 PM

Activities: Schedule your most demanding, focused, or creative tasks and important meetings during this peak energy period.

Nutrition: Enjoy a balanced lunch that includes lean proteins, healthy fats, and complex carbohydrates. Grilled chicken or tofu with greens and roasted vegetables, a hearty salad with avocado and salmon, or whole-grain bread with grilled chicken, hummus, and veggies are great options.

Hydration: Sip on water throughout this time with slices of lemon or cucumber for cell health and energy.

Foods:

+ Berries (strawberries, raspberries, blueberries)
+ Hydrating fruits (cherries, oranges, peaches, apricots)
+ Tomatoes, peppers
+ Tropical fruits (pineapple, mango, papaya)
+ Leafy greens (romaine lettuce, spinach, arugula, basil)
+ Cucumbers, melons (watermelon, cantaloupe)
+ Zucchini, summer squash

Flavors:

+ Bitter foods like broccoli or artichokes
+ Spicy foods such as chili peppers and ginger can help stimulate circulation

Harvest/Earth (Afternoon and Early Evening): 2:00 PM–7:00 PM

Activities: Tie up loose ends from the day, and focus on tasks that require organization and attention to detail. Check in with family and report on your day. Finish up everything so your mind can be prepared for resting.

Nutrition: Enjoy a light and nutritious dinner that is easy to digest and won't interfere with your sleep. Consider options like grilled fish with steamed vegetables, a leafy green salad with lean protein, or a hearty vegetable soup with whole-grain bread.

Foods:

- ✦ Root vegetables (carrots, sweet potatoes, beets)
- ✦ Squashes (acorn and butternut squash, pumpkin)
- ✦ Grains (rice, oats, quinoa, barley, quinoa, amaranth)
- ✦ Legumes (pinto beans, lentils, chickpeas, adzuki beans)
- ✦ Nuts and seeds (almonds, pumpkin seeds, pecans)
- ✦ Fruits with a sweet taste (apples, pears, dates, figs)
- ✦ Maple syrup, honey
- ✦ Whole grains

Flavors:

- ✦ Sweet foods like sweet potatoes, carrots, and grains
- ✦ Slightly spicy foods like ginger and cinnamon to aid digestion

Reflection: Reflect on your achievements and successes from the day, celebrate your progress and adjust priorities and set realistic goals for the remainder of the day.

Fall/Air (Evening): 7:00 PM–11:00 PM

Activities: Shift your focus to less demanding tasks. Read a book, practice gentle yoga, take a walk, or listen to calming music.

Snacking: If you need to snack, choose light foods that are easy to digest like Greek yogurt with berries, an apple and two dates, or sliced veggies with hummus.

Foods:

- ✦ White vegetables (cauliflower, cabbage, onions, mushrooms, beans)
- ✦ Pungent vegetables (garlic, ginger, onions, radishes)
- ✦ Spices (ginger, cinnamon, cloves)
- ✦ Warming fruits (pears, apples, grapes, pomegranates)
- ✦ Nuts and seeds (almonds, walnuts)
- ✦ White fish

Flavors:

✦ Garlic, onions, and radishes to help clear the lungs and promote healthy digestion.

✦ Spices like ginger, cinnamon, and cloves for warmth and vitality.

Relaxation: Dim the lights, turn off electronic devices, and take a warm bath or drink a cup of hot chamomile tea to tell your body it's time to wind down.

Winter/Water (Nighttime and Early Morning): 11:00 PM–5:00 AM

Activities: Unplug from screens and technology at least an hour before bedtime, read a book, practice gentle yoga or meditation, or journal about your day.

Nutrition:

1. Eating should be minimal or completely avoided close to bedtime, as food being digested can disrupt your sleep, which will leave you feeling sluggish in the morning.
2. If you need to eat something, stick to a broth based soup, banana, or handful of berries.

Foods:

✦ Miso soup
✦ Bone broth
✦ Blackberries

Flavors:

✦ Salty and umami foods like seaweed, miso, and sea salt

Sleep Hygiene: Create a restful sleep environment by ensuring your bedroom is dark, quiet, and cool. Remove all electronics from the room to eliminate EMFs that could disturb your cellular signaling.

Eating and Living with the Seasons

When Elaine first walked into my office, she was an emotional wreck, overwhelmed by conflicting health and nutrition advice. Her health had worsened since a childhood accident at thirteen, resulting in a root canal that years later raised concerns of infection. Struggling with rheumatoid arthritis, Elaine worried the infected tooth could be worsening her symptoms. A cone beam CT scan confirmed her fears, and she decided to replace the tooth with a ceramic dental implant. This process would require surgery, and she was worried she wouldn't heal well. Determined to prepare her body, she delved into nutrition research, only to find more contradictions. Each day brought new, conflicting dietary advice, leaving her unsure about what to eat and when to eat it.

Once I introduced her to the Cell Well model, Elaine realized that it was more important to understand the natural rhythms of her own body than to rely on the fluctuating trends she heard about from friends or read about on social media or the internet. With this newfound understanding, Elaine's daily routine transformed into predictable, well-timed meals and activities that aligned with the natural needs of her cells and body. After her surgery, Elaine continued to follow these Seasons of the Day cycles and was surprised by how easy her recovery was: she had little to no pain and almost no swelling in her mouth. But what truly shocked Elaine was the resolution of many of her arthritis symptoms. Her stiff and swollen fingers flexed a little further, and her knees and hips were less achy every day. Elaine realized she had found a new lifestyle that would keep her and her cells well.

Cell Well Body Clock

A concept in traditional Chinese medicine called the body clock outlines the flow of energy through different organs at specific times of the day. This cycle is believed to optimize the functioning of each organ and enhance overall health. This concept inspired the Cell Well Body Clock. Here's a breakdown of the Cell Well Body Clock and the organs associated with each time period and Season of the Day.

Body Clock

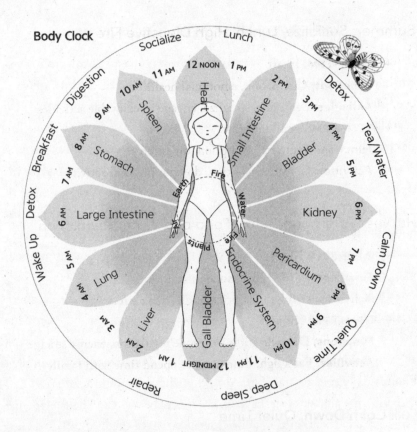

Spring: Wake Up Detox, Breakfast, Early Digestion

+ **5 AM–7 AM:** Large intestine

  Functions: Elimination, detoxification

  Activities: Drink water, have bowel movements, eat a light breakfast

+ **7 AM–9 AM:** Stomach

  Functions: Digestion, nutrient absorption

  Activities: Eat a hearty breakfast, avoid stress, engage in physical activities

+ **9 AM–11 AM:** Spleen

  Functions: Digestion, energy production, immune support

  Activities: Focus on work or productive tasks, eat a light snack

Summer: Socialize, Lunch, High Digestive Fire

✦ **11 AM–1 PM:** Heart
   Functions: Circulation, emotional health
   Activities: Eat lunch, socialize, engage in enjoyable activities
✦ **1 PM–3 PM:** Small intestine
   Functions: Nutrient absorption, digestion
   Activities: Continue working, do light physical activity

Harvest: Afternoon Detox, Food and Water Regulation

✦ **3 PM–5 PM:** Bladder
   Functions: Fluid regulation, detoxification
   Activities: Drink fluids, stretch, do light exercise
✦ **5 PM–7 PM:** Kidney
   Functions: Detoxification, hormone regulation, energy storage
   Activities: Eat a light dinner, relax, spend time with family

Fall: Calm Down, Quiet Time

✦ **7 PM–9 PM:** Pericardium
   Functions: Circulation, emotional balance
   Activities: Relax, do light reading, meditate, enjoy hobbies
✦ **9 PM–11 PM:** Endocrine system
   Functions: Regulation of water metabolism, temperature balance
   Activities: Prepare for sleep, engage in calming activities

Winter: Deep Sleep, Repair

✦ **11 PM–1 AM:** Gallbladder
   Functions: Digestion of fats, decision making
   Activities: Sleep, allow the body to rest and rejuvenate

+ **1 AM–3 AM:** Liver
  Functions: Detoxification, blood filtration, emotional processing
  Activities: Sleep deeply as the body undergoes detoxification and repair
+ **3 AM–5 AM:** Lung
  Functions: Respiration, immune system
  Activities: Do breathing exercises, stretch gently, meditate

Using the Seasons of the Day and the Cell Well Body Clock information, as well as the Seasons guides found in chapter 10, you can create a personalized plan for wellness.

CHAPTER 13

The Cell Well Formula!

It's time to learn about Cell Well Formulas.

Learning to navigate the Cell Well model and master the art of cellular health is similar to learning to ride a bike. I remember my very first bike. It was red, had a long banana-shaped seat, and had white plastic streamers coming out of the end of each handlebar. I loved that bike, and I was terrified yet excited to straddle it for the very first time. The seat felt enormous, the handlebars wide, and the very thought of balancing on those two wheels seemed impossible, but with my dad's help, I was soon riding up and down the street.

Learning to make the choices that will keep your cells well—and developing the strength, discipline, and stamina to keep going on the path—is just like riding a bicycle! It takes courage, practice, perseverance, and a little help. And, just like riding a bicycle, once you know how to keep your cells well, you'll never forget.

Cell Well Formulas

Cell Well Formulas are simple ways to combine nutrition, exercise, and lifestyle choices to proactively give your cells what they need to stay well and have the energy they need in any Season and at any time of day. To help you grasp the concept of Cell Well Formulas, I will share stories based on issues faced by patients in my practice and the Cell Well Formulas they used to overcome their challenges. Keep in mind that these examples demonstrate how to apply the Elements and Seasons, rather than serving as exact prescriptions for you. Use them as guides to understand how incorporating the Cell Well model into your life can be systematic and seamless.

Sarah's Spring/Plants Cell Well Formula

Sarah was struggling with painful numbness in her hands. The numbness interfered with simple tasks like blow-drying her hair or typing on her computer, and she woke up multiple times a night in tears from the pain. Doctors suggested surgery for carpal tunnel, but Sarah couldn't afford the time off work. Desperate to find a solution, she came to see me to find out if her old mercury fillings could be contributing to the numbness. As we talked, Sarah shared more symptoms, including a growing sensitivity to foods like dairy, gluten, corn, and more.

During Sarah's dental exam, I discovered five old mercury fillings. Following SMART (Safe Mercury Amalgam Removal Technique) safety protocols, she had them removed. We discussed how mercury could affect her cells, particularly the security of her liver and its cell signaling pathways. I suggested that Sarah try out the Spring/Plants Cell Well Formula, and she agreed.

By supporting her liver with specific foods and supplements and the activities listed below, Sarah began using the Cell Well model to rid her body of mercury and return her cells to wellness.[275]

Supply

1. Breakfast: Cell Well Green Smoothie, or two scrambled eggs cooked with onions and garlic.
2. Lunch: Salad with mixed greens, baby carrots, cherry tomatoes, avocado, and leftover grilled salmon or chicken, or a sandwich with the same vegetables and protein.

3. Dinner: Chicken breast or white fish seasoned with herbs and served with roasted broccoli and cauliflower.

4. Drink: Water that has gone through a reverse osmosis filter and had minerals added back.

Support and Secure

Sarah added the following supplements to her wellness regimen:

1. **Milk thistle:** 150–300 mg of standardized milk thistle extract daily for liver health and detoxification.

2. **N-acetylcysteine (NAC):** 600–1200 mg of NAC daily for detoxification.

Signal

To help strengthen cell signaling, Sarah incorporated the following activities into her schedule:

1. Movement: A moderate, one- to three-mile walk every day.

2. Yoga: Spring/Plants yoga poses three times a week in the evening while getting ready for bed.

3. Brush: Using a skin brush after getting out of the shower.

Within a month of removing the fillings and incorporating the Spring/Plants Cell Well Formula, Sarah's numbness vanished—no further surgery required. That was when she realized her symptoms had been her cells telling her what they needed to be well. The mercury in her fillings had clogged her liver, causing inflammation that affected every cell in her body, including the channels the blood vessels and nerves passed through when going to her hands. This channel (the carpal tunnel) was swollen, cutting off both blood supply and cell signals, leading to numbness. Detoxifying and supporting her liver led to decreased inflammation and less swelling and eliminated the pain Sarah had been experiencing.[276] With the Cell Well model, Sarah had what she needed to understand and support her body's natural healing processes.

Jodi's Summer/Fire Cell Well Formula

Jodi was a long-time patient of mine and always the picture of health. She had run fifty marathons by the age of fifty, and her life was full of early morning running, cycling, and training for triathlon races. Yet beneath this veneer of robust health, her cells were experiencing a silent problem that threatened to halt her racing and even her life.

During a routine dental checkup, Jodi shared a terrifying experience she'd had recently. For years, Jodi had been seeing "stars" during intense runs. Being in good shape, and assuming herself to be in good health, Jodi had brushed these symptoms off as signs of fatigue. However, her condition had recently taken a frightening turn. On a crisp morning, during a run with friends, an invisible weight seemed to clamp tightly around Jodi's head. The world spun wildly, forcing her to stop and sit by the roadside, her breath ragged and heartbeat erratic. Insisting her friends continue, Jodi attempted to cross the street to a nearby church but passed out cold on the asphalt halfway across the road.

A concerned motorist found Jodi unconscious and immediately called an ambulance. In the hospital, Jodi's heart stopped and restarted twice, terrifying both her family and the medical professionals around her. The attending doctor told her she had simply worn her heart out and that she needed a procedure called an ablation. The ablation would restore a normal rhythm to her heart, like fixing a short circuit in an electrical system.

When Jodi visited my office, she was waiting for the ablation and worried that her heart might give out before she could make it to the scheduled appointment. When I learned about her condition, I began by establishing a rigorous oral hygiene regimen for Jodi. With a weakened heart, the risk of bacteria from her mouth infecting her heart was too high. Next, we discussed the role of nutrition in Jodi's heart health. Every bite of food she took could be a step toward healing. Determined to avoid further scares, Jodi started following a Summer/Fire Cell Well Formula, combining healing red and orange foods with a more moderate exercise program and heart-healthy herbs to nurture her heart at the cellular level.

Once Jodi started on this Formula, she began to see improvements in her health in just a few weeks. Her energy returned, and her mind was clearer than it had been in months. Jodi felt much better, but her husband, haunted by the memory of her heart stopping in the hospital, pressed for her to continue with the scheduled ablation. On the day of the procedure, however, what the doctors found—or rather did not find—was astonishing. There was nothing to correct; Jodi's heart had healed itself. It had responded to Jodi's new nutrition and lifestyle changes. The doctors didn't proceed with the surgery and simply sent Jodi home to continue doing what she was doing to rebuild her cells and heart. Her return to health is not just a medical success but a Cell Well triumph!

Supply

1. Breakfast: Oatmeal with walnuts, blueberries, sliced strawberries, and a touch of honey.
2. Lunch: Whole grain toast with Tomato Cucumber Bruschetta and grilled salmon.
3. Dinner: Savory Crockpot Lentil Stew served over rice.
4. Avoid: Spicy, greasy, and sugary foods.

Support and Secure

Jodi supplemented her diet with:

1. **Omega-3 fatty acids:** 1,000–2,000 mg daily to reduce inflammation.
2. **Curcumin:** 500 mg twice daily to fight inflammation.
3. **Ginger:** 500 mg daily to help with digestion and inflammation.
4. **Probiotics:** Daily to help with overall immunity and inflammation management.

Signal

To help strengthen cell signaling, Jodi added the following activities to her day:

1. Yoga: Summer/Fire yoga poses to improve circulation and reduce inflammation.
2. Movement: Moderate exercise, such as walking or swimming for thirty minutes a day in the morning or evening. Avoid intense exercise in the heat of the day.
3. Drink: Naturally electrolyte-rich beverages like coconut water, or add a pinch of salt and a squeeze of lemon to water.
4. Avoid: Removing all electronics, including charging devices, from her bedroom to eliminate EMFs at night.

Sameer's Harvest/Earth Cell Well Formula

Sameer had been counting the days until he could graduate with his master's degree in accounting and start his long-awaited new job as an accountant at Ernst and Young, one of the "Big Four" accounting firms. His excitement was mixed with understandable anxiety about the pressure of this next step. This was a significant milestone. However, five weeks before he was contracted to start, he got very sick.

At first, his symptoms seemed innocent enough: extreme fatigue, a sore throat, and swollen lymph nodes, all of which he thought could be chalked up to pre-job anxiety. He and his wife Nisha tried all the quick fix remedies they could find on the internet, hoping for a speedy recovery. But Sameer's condition only worsened. Not only did he have debilitating fatigue and a sore throat, but he also developed unusual little red spots, like tiny bruises, on the inside of his cheeks and gums and across the roof of his mouth. To compound his misery, a severe outbreak of cold sores erupted on Sameer's lips.

Concerned, Sameer and Nisha visited my office. Noting the sore throat and swollen lips, I suspected a viral infection far more serious than stress or anxiety and recommended that he see a doctor. Following my advice, Sameer visited his family doctor, who diagnosed him with infectious mononucleosis, commonly known as mono. Mono, caused by the Epstein-Barr virus, primarily spreads through saliva and is known for inducing symptoms like fever, sore throat, swollen lymph nodes, and fatigue. More critically for

Sameer, the virus had caused his spleen to swell, putting him at risk for a ruptured spleen, a potentially life-threatening complication.

His doctor recommended that Sameer postpone his start date at work, but he was scared that if he postponed, he would lose the position, a highly coveted spot that many other new graduates would be happy to fill. Unsure of what to do next, Nisha reached out to me for additional guidance on how they could speed up his recovery. Together, we planned out a Harvest/ Earth Cell Well Formula for Sameer to focus on nutrition, and we chose targeted supplements to boost Sameer's immune system and help his cells heal. This wasn't just about managing his symptoms. It was about nurturing his body at a cellular level.

As Sameer's start date neared, he had recovered about 70 percent of his normal health. His throat was no longer sore, the cold sores and red spots in his mouth had resolved, and his energy levels were returning. Sameer wasn't fully recovered, but he was well enough to make this new start feasible. With a well-stocked refrigerator and supplement cupboard, and support from his wife, he embarked on this new phase of life.

Supply

1. Breakfast: Oatmeal topped with sliced strawberries, chopped walnuts, and a drizzle of honey. Can add Greek yogurt or almond milk for even more protein.
2. Lunch: Salad with rice, roasted vegetables, lettuce, sliced red peppers, and nitrate-free deli chicken.
3. Dinner: Baked salmon with Oven-Roasted Broccoli and rice pilaf.
4. Snacks: Apples with almond butter, carrot sticks with hummus, or a handful of mixed nuts and seeds.

Support and Secure

Sameer supplemented his diet with:

1. **Vitamin C:** 1,000–2,000 mg of vitamin C per day to boost the immune system.

2. **Zinc:** 15–30 mg per day of zinc gluconate or zinc citrate for immune strength and healing.
3. **Vitamin D3:** 1,000–2,000 IU per day of vitamin D3 for immune strength.
4. **Herbal Remedies:** Echinacea, astragalus, and licorice root supplements to aid in recovery from the viral infection.

Signal

To help strengthen cell signaling, Sameer added the following activities to his schedule:

1. Rest: Avoiding overexertion so the body can heal.
2. Earthing: Touching the earth for at least twenty minutes per day (ex: walking barefoot outside, sitting on the lawn).
3. Yoga: Harvest/Earth earth yoga poses three times a week.
4. Avoid: Minimizing time on the computer and phone and using EMF protection devices at work.

Yuna's Fall/Air Cell Well Formula

Yuna was meticulous about her dental hygiene, which was why she became alarmed when a back molar became sensitive. Hoping for a simple explanation and a quick fix, she made an appointment at my dental office. I examined her teeth and took traditional dental X-rays, but everything appeared normal—no cavities, no decay, no obvious reason for her discomfort. Still, something seemed off, so I decided to take a cone beam CT scan to get a clearer picture. As the scan loaded on the screen, I was shocked, not by the condition of her tooth (which was fine), but by something far more concerning. Yuna's airway was nearly completely closed. It looked like she was suffocating!

I asked about her sleeping habits, which opened the door to a flood of frustrations she had been dealing with for years. Yuna revealed that she had struggled tremendously with sleeping, relying on pharmaceutical aids for over a decade without much real relief. Recently, even these aids had stopped working, subjecting her to sleepless nights that left her brain foggy and her body exhausted during the day. All this had also left her with a caffeine dependency, a chronic dry cough, and an erratic heartbeat. Yuna felt like her life was a nonstop cycle of fatigue and frustration, with no end in sight. She was elated when we told her that her insomnia was something that a Cell Well formula and specialized dental care could help with.

Because of inflammation in her cells and body due in part to some of her diet choices, Yuna's throat was often clogged with mucus and the tissue in the back of her mouth was swollen, sagging into her throat and blocking off the flow of air. To correct the problem and improve her sleep, I suggested a Cell Well formula focused on decreasing mucus and inflammation and clearing out her cells, along with a straightforward laser procedure that could shrink the blocking tissue and open her airway. The combination of these two things could potentially transform her sleep quality—and her life. Yuna eagerly asked if she could get started immediately. We scheduled her first laser session that day and gave her instruction for her Fall/Air Cell Well Formula to boost her cell health and breathing.

After the first month, Yuna reported she had been going to sleep easier at night but was still waking frequently. The amazing transformation came after her second month. She was sleeping regularly again, her heart rhythm had normalized, and she was free from the constant colds that had plagued her before. As it turned out, the sensitivity in her molar was due to her clenching her teeth at night in an unconscious effort to open her blocked airway. With her inflammation down and healthier cells, her sleeping was restored, the clenching stopped, and Yuna's tooth sensitivity disappeared.

More importantly, with every breath she took, Yuna was filling her cells with the oxygen they needed to create energy and be well.

Supply

1. Breakfast: Oatmeal with sliced pears and a sprinkle of ground flaxseed.
2. Lunch: Cauliflower rice bowl or salad with radishes.
3. Dinner: Baked salmon with steamed spinach and a side of rice.
4. Avoid: Dairy and bananas, which can produce mucus.

Support and Secure

Yuna supplemented her diet with:

1. **Fish oil:** 1,000–2,000 mg daily to reduce inflammation.
2. **Vitamin C:** 500–1,000 mg daily to increase immune function.
3. **Probiotics:** Daily to support gut and lung health.

Signal

To help strengthen cell signaling, Yuna incorporated the following activities into her life:

1. Breathing exercises to strengthen the lungs.
2. Movement: Moderate exercise, such as walking or swimming, for thirty minutes a day in the morning or evening.
3. Avoid: Smoking and exposure to pollutants, as well as drafts and cold wind.

Matteo's Winter/Water Cell Well Formula

When Matteo began to experience recurrent kidney stones, along with the accompanying episodes of extreme pain, he went through a handful of treatments and got many opinions, but no one he spoke to could pinpoint the cause. However, during his visit to my office, one of my hygienists noticed he had an unusual amount of hardened tartar on his teeth and his gums were infected around the buildup. As we talked about cause for the buildup and infection, a possible solution for the buildup and his kidney stones emerged.

Matteo worked as a marketing director for multiple small companies. His job was to put out marketing fires for these companies, and he sat indoors, at his computer, for sixty or more hours a week. When working, he would go hours, sometimes days, without eating or drinking anything other than sugary drinks and packaged snack foods. These foods were high in sugar and salt and deficient in vitamins and minerals. Matteo also rarely saw the sun, so his vitamin D levels were very low. I explained to Matteo that his body and cells were trying to balance the high sugar and salt in his snack food diet, and to do that, they had to get rid of minerals in the cells, including calcium. The kidneys and saliva have the job of removing that excess calcium, and if they don't have the help of other minerals like magnesium and vitamins like D3 and K2, that calcium will form mineral buildup in the kidneys, forming stones, and other places in the body, including tartar on the teeth. We cleaned the tartar and sent Matteo home with a Winter/Water Cell Well Formula, hoping to prevent more mineral buildup from forming in his body.

Three months later Matteo returned to my office for a followup cleaning and couldn't wait to talk to me. Desperate for help, he had been following his Cell Well formula exactly. Not only did he have much less tartar to clean off his teeth, he hadn't had any kidney problems at all. Hopeful this was a long-term answer, he had changed his eating and working schedule to help give his cells what they needed to stay well. Cleaning up his diet and getting more sunshine and movement likely helped restore Matteo's cellular environment to normal, allowing his body to utilize calcium rather than try to get rid of it. When I saw Matteo for his next cleaning appointment, Matteo reported continued improvements in his kidney health and was optimistic about his future wellness.

Supply

1. Breakfast: Hot cooked millet or oats with blackberries and blueberries, 8 ounces of celery juice or grapefruit juice, alternating days.
2. Lunch: Six-Can Chili or salad with black beans and kidney beans.
3. Dinner: Miso Glazed Salmon.
4. Snack: Sliced cucumbers and Chia Lime Refresher.

Support and Secure

Stuart supplemented his diet with:

1. **Fish oil:** 1,000–2,000 mg daily to reduce inflammation.
2. **Vitamin D3/K2:** 1,000–2,000 IU daily of vitamin D3 and 100–200 mcg daily of vitamin K2. Helps regulate mineral levels in the cells.
3. **Magnesium:** 300–400 mg of magnesium daily to protect against stone formation.

Signal

To help strengthen cell signaling, Matteo incorporated the following activities into his life:

1. Hydration: Eight to ten glasses of water daily, and more if he was very active.
2. Movement: A fifteen-minute walk outside every day for a natural dose of vitamin D and Winter/Water yoga poses in the evening before bed.
3. Food: Warm or hot foods and beverages to support internal warmth and aid digestion.

Road Map to Wellness

Now that you know how to map out your day to follow the Seasons, and you see how Cell Well Formulas are built, it's time to assess where you are now, build your Personal Cell Well Formula, and get going!

Step 1: Assess your starting Season with the Seasons of Wellness Assessment.

Step 2: Use the Seasons Snapshot to verify that your symptoms correlate with that season.

Step 3: Use the Seasons guides to create your own Cell Well Formula. Learn about the food, supplement, and lifestyle changes that will be especially beneficial for you.

Step 4: Choose one recommendation in your Formula to start with.

Step 5: Begin following Seasons of the Day recommendations to bring you closer to wellness every day.

Step 6: Move at your own pace through your Cell Well Formula, seeking support from health care practitioners that combine traditional and modern medicine.

Your Personal Cell Well Formula

Use the steps listed above and the blank template below to design your own Cell Well Formula. You can find information about foods, supplement/ herbal, and lifestyle recommendations for each Season in chapter 10.

Starting Season:

Starting Symptoms:

Supply

Foods to try:

+ Breakfast:
+ Lunch:
+ Dinner:
+ Snacks:

Support and Secure

Supplement or herbal recommendations to try:

Signal

Lifestyle recommendations to try:

Your Wellness Journey Has Begun

Having faith in your cells and supporting them with the right tools can make a significant difference in your health, lifespan, healthspan, and wellness. As you've journeyed through this book, you have traveled from the microscopic realm of cells to the macrocosm of the grand tapestry of the earth's Elements and Seasons. You have learned that your organs and their systems are intricately woven from billions of interconnected cells, and that for you to be well, each of those cells needs to be well.

Each day, your cells face many challenges, from environmental toxins to emotional stressors, each leaving an indelible epigenetic imprint on your cellular blueprint epigenetically. You've learned that there are benefits and limitations in both modern Western medicine and traditional medicine and that combining approaches holds the key to unlocking the full potential of cellular and whole-body wellness.

The Cell Well model, with its emphasis on supplying, supporting, securing, and signaling in your cells, has proven time and again to be effective in promoting wellness and preventing illness. By understanding and applying the principles and practices you've learned here, you too can keep your cells well and enjoy a healthier, more vibrant life. Plants feed your body and cells. Earth delivers electrons and minerals to your cells. Water carries nutrients to your cells and eliminates toxic wastes. Fire ignites your energy through electrons and cell signals, and air supercharges each cell's energy production. These Elements work in harmony with the natural cyclical rhythms of the earth and your body. From the awakening of spring to the abundance of summer, the bringing in of harvest, letting go of fall, and the introspection of winter, each season has its own purpose that adds to wellness.

Now that you understand how your cells work and how to use the Elements and Seasons, you are ready to craft your own Personal Wellness Formula—a blend of nourishment, movement, and intentional practices tailored to your unique cellular and body-wide needs. You don't need to be a passive observer on your wellness journey. You have everything you need to be an active participant in life. Each cell within you carries the blueprint, wisdom, resilience, and innate capacity for healing and transformation.

Thank you for taking care of your cells and yourself. You deserve to be, and will be, well.

APPENDIX 1

Seasonal Recipes

Included here are all the recipes listed in *Living Well with Dr. Michelle* by Season/Element. (Everything in this appendix can also be found at www.resources.livingwellbook.com.)

Seasonal Recipe Index

Spring/Plants Recipes

SPRING/PLANTS RECIPES

Cell Well Green Smoothie

This recipe can be adapted by using any combination of greens and fruit that you have available or are in season where you live. Seasonal fruits and greens are always higher in nutritional value than those that are out of season.

- 1 cup water
- 1 tablespoon flax oil
- 3 cups fresh greens (spinach, kale, or lettuce)
- 1 banana, orange, or apple, cut into quarters
- 1 cup frozen berries
- 1 teaspoon honey (optional)
- 1 tablet calcium lactate to counteract the oxalates in the greens (optional)

Step 1. Blend water, flax oil, and greens for 1 minute.

Step 2. Add fruit and tablet if desired. Blend until smooth, 1 additional minute.

Step 3. Add honey as needed for taste.

Yield: 1–2 servings

Morning Detox Smoothie

This smoothie is a tasty way to help your cells detox during the spring hours of the morning. Antioxidants in the lemon juice and apple, B vitamins and minerals in the greens, omega-3 fatty acids in the chia seeds, and other plant chemicals and fiber in the ginger and cucumber.

- 1 cup fresh spinach
- 1 small cucumber, quartered
- 1 apple, quartered
- 1 tablespoon lemon juice
- 1 tablespoon chia seeds
- ½ inch piece of fresh ginger root, diced
- 1-1 ½ cups of coconut water or filtered water
- A few leaves of fresh mint (optional)
- Honey or liquid stevia (optional)
- 1 tablet calcium lactate to counteract the oxalates in the greens (optional)

Step 1. In a blender combine the spinach, cucumber, apple, lemon juice, chia seeds, ginger, and mint leaves and tablets if desired.

Step 2. Pour in the coconut water or filtered water.

Step 3. Blend until smooth. If it's too thick, add more liquid.

Step 4. Taste for sweetness and add honey or a few drops of liquid stevia to taste.

Yield: 1 serving

Chia Lime Refresher

This recipe is patterned after a drink used by the Tarahumara people in Mexico to boost endurance and energy. Also known as "chia fresca," it provides many benefits to your cells, including hydration, essential nutrients (omega-3 fatty acids, protein, fiber, antioxidants, vitamins, and minerals), natural electrolytes (vitamin C and potassium), and a natural source of carbohydrates and sugars for energy. Try it as your morning "let's get going" drink!

- 16 ounces of filtered water
- 1 tablespoon dry chia seeds
- 2 teaspoons lime juice
- 1 teaspoon honey (optional)

Step 1. Combine water, chia seeds, lime juice, and honey and stir to blend.

Step 2. Let sit for five minutes.

Step 3. Stir again and let sit for as long as you like. The more it sits, the more gel-like the seeds and water become.

Yield: 1 serving

Well Liver Tea

Herbal tea recipes list ingredients either by specific amount or by "parts." This recipe is listed in parts so you can premake a bulk amount or make just enough for a few servings.

- 1 part rosehips
- 1 part dried burdock root
- 2 parts milk thistle seed
- 2 parts holy basil
- 2 parts dried dandelion root

Step 1. Add the dried herbs to a glass storage jar or container with a tight lid.

Step 2. Gently shake to blend the herbs. Label and date with herbs used and their amounts. Store indefinitely.

Step 3. To use the tea mixture, place 2 tablespoons in a reusable tea bag or tea strainer.

Step 4. Cover with 1 quart boiling water.

Step 5. Allow to steep for 8 to 10 minutes.

Step 6. Strain herbs, sweeten to taste, and enjoy.

Recipe Note: You can enjoy this cold, pouring pre-sweetened tea over a glass of ice. You can also make a larger batch of this tea and store in the fridge for up to 3 days.

Yield: 2 servings (per 2 tablespoons tea blend)

Oven-Roasted Broccoli

Broccoli is good for detoxing your cells because of its sulfur content. You can substitute other vegetables in the same family in this recipe, such as cauliflower and cabbage.

- 1 large head (12 oz) broccoli florets
- 1 tablespoon extra virgin olive oil
- 1 teaspoon cumin
- ½ teaspoon garlic powder
- ½ teaspoon salt
- ⅛ teaspoon freshly ground black pepper

Step 1. Preheat the oven to 400°F.

Step 2. Place the broccoli florets into a bowl and toss with the olive oil and spices.

Step 3. Spread evenly on a 13 x 18-inch baking sheet.

Step 4. Roast 15 to 22 minutes or until browned around the edges.

Yield: 2–4 servings

Melt-in-Your-Mouth Cauliflower

This cauliflower is melt-in-your-mouth delicious, full of detoxing sulfur, healthy fats, and salt, a natural electrolyte.

- 1 medium head (24 oz) cauliflower
- 2 cups water
- 1 teaspoon salt
- 2 tablespoons olive oil
- 1 tablespoon kosher salt

Step 1. Preheat the oven to 425°F.

Step 2. Wash the cauliflower, remove any leaves, and cut the bottom of the stem.

Step 3. Put the whole head in a pan with a lid. Add the water and 1 teaspoon salt.

Step 4. Cover and bring to a boil. Boil for 10 minutes.

Step 5. Lift out of the water and place on a 13 x 18-inch baking sheet. Pour the olive oil over the top, and sprinkle on the kosher salt.

Step 6. Bake for 24 minutes, until browned on top. Turn once while cooking.

Yield: 4–6 servings

Lemonade Beet Salad

This beet salad is so tasty even the kids will love it. Try using a yellow and a red beet for added color.

- 2 large raw beets, washed (and peeled if skin is tough)
- 1 tablespoon olive oil
- 2 tablespoons lemon juice
- 1 teaspoon honey
- ¼ teaspoon salt

Step 1. Wash and peel beets. Grate on a large size grater or use a spiralizer to cut into thin strands.

Step 2. Toss with other ingredients. Taste for sweetness and add more honey if desired.

Step 3. Let sit for 5 minutes to let flavors blend before serving.

Yield: 4 servings

Six-Can Chili

This recipe comes together in five minutes and can be cooked in a slow cooker or on the stovetop. Bonus: the beans provide complex carbohydrates for energy!

- 1 can (28 oz) diced tomatoes
- 1 can (15 oz) chili beans
- 1 can (15 oz each) garbanzo beans, pinto beans, and black beans, drained
- 1 can (4 oz) chopped green chiles
- 3 teaspoons chili powder
- 1 teaspoon cumin
- 1 teaspoon oregano
- ½ teaspoon salt

Toppings
- Shredded cheese
- Tortilla chips
- Avocado
- Shredded lettuce

Step 1. Combine all ingredients in a slow cooker and cook for 6–8 hours on low, or put in a pan on the stove and cook for 20 minutes until flavors are blended.

Step 2. Put the shredded lettuce in a bowl and add the chili and toppings.

Yield: 8 servings

Crockpot Spaghetti Sauce

Canned pasta sauces are often full of sugar and other things I don't want to add to my dinner. This tomato-and-herb-filled version is so much tastier and nutritious, I never buy the cans anymore. Start this in the crockpot before the day gets crazy and you will have a delicious dinner just when you need it.

- 1 pound (16 oz) ground beef
- 1 cup frozen green peppers and onions
- 2 teaspoons garlic, minced (fresh or from a jar)
- 3 cans (15 oz each) diced tomatoes
- 2 cans (8 oz each) tomato sauce
- 1 can (6 oz) tomato paste
- 2 tablespoons honey
- 3 teaspoons Italian seasoning
- 1 teaspoon salt
- Regular or gluten-free noodles

Step 1. Brown the ground beef, peppers, and onions together in a pan. Add to the crockpot, along with all other ingredients except the noodles.

Step 2. Cook on low for 6–8 hours

Step 3. Cook the noodles as instructed on the package.

Step 4. Serve sauce over cooked noodles.

Yield: 8 servings

One-Pan Frittata

On my Living Well homestead, we have fresh vegetables and eggs available all through the summer. Aiming to use everything we produce, I came up with this easy, thrown-together-quickly meal to use our bounty.

- 2–3 cups mixed veggies, chopped (frozen or fresh)
- 1 tablespoon coconut oil
- 9 eggs
- 1 teaspoon salt
- 1 teaspoon Italian seasoning
- ½ cup feta cheese

Step 1. Sauté mixed veggies in coconut oil until barely tender. Remove half from pan and set aside.

Step 2. Whisk eggs and seasonings together in a bowl and pour over top of veggies in pan. Cook until set.

Step 3. Add remaining veggies back on top of eggs. Sprinkle with cheese.

Step 4. Put under broiler for 2–3 min until browned.

Yield: 4–6 servings

Crockpot Enchilada Casserole

I love Mexican-inspired food because it's an easy way to sneak plants into a meal! This casserole saves you the time of rolling individual enchiladas. I often make it from leftovers from another meal.

- 1 pound (16 oz) ground beef (optional for vegetarian)
- ½ cup onion, chopped (fresh or frozen)
- ½ teaspoon garlic, minced (fresh or from a jar)
- ½ teaspoon salt
- ½ teaspoon pepper
- 3 cups frozen Mexican-style mixed vegetables (corn, red peppers, onions, tomatoes)
- 1 can (15 oz) black beans, drained
- 12 corn or grain-free tortillas
- 1 can (19 oz) red or green enchilada sauce
- 2 cups shredded cheddar cheese
- Shredded lettuce

Step 1. Brown ground beef, onion, and garlic together with salt and pepper in a skillet over medium heat.

Step 2. Combine frozen mixed vegetables with the black beans in a bowl.

Step 3. Break up 3 tortillas into large pieces and spread on the bottom of the crockpot.

Step 4. Put 1/3 of the enchilada sauce over the tortillas, top with 1/3 of the ground beef mixture, then 1/3 of the veggies and beans, and top with 1/3 of the cheese.

Step 5. Repeat by making another layer of 3 more tortillas, then 1/3 of the sauce, followed by meat, veggies, and beans, and top with cheese.

Step 6. Repeat one more time using the last 1/3 of all the ingredients for the last layer and end with 3 tortillas broken into pieces on the top.

Step 7. Cover and cook on low 6–8 hours. Serve with shredded lettuce.

Yield: 6–8 servings

Weekend Pulled Chicken

This recipe makes a great meal that combines convenience foods with whole foods in a way that is nutritious and delicious. It is an easy crowd favorite that can be put together in minutes.

- 2 pounds chicken breasts
- ½ of a 15-ounce bottle of zesty Italian dressing
- ½ tablespoon minced garlic (fresh or from a jar)
- ½ tablespoon chili powder
- ½ tablespoon ground cumin
- Shredded lettuce
- Shredded cheese
- Corn tortillas

Step 1. Place chicken, dressing, and spices in a crock pot.

Step 2. Cook on high 5–6 hours or on low for 8 hours.

Step 3. When it is done cooking and tender, remove the chicken to a plate and shred it with two forks.

Step 4. Add the chicken back to the liquid left in the crockpot and stir together.

Step 5. Serve with lettuce, cheese, and tortillas as desired.

Yield: 8 servings

Guacamole

This is a simple Cell Well treat everyone loves!

- 2 large avocados, pits removed
- ¼ cup bottled salsa
- 1 lime, juiced (2 tablespoons)
- ¼ teaspoon salt

Step 1. Combine all ingredients in a bowl and mash with a potato masher or fork.

Yield: 8 servings

Tastes Like Scratch Black Beans

Beans provide nutrients that your appestat is looking for. This quick treatment can turn a can of plain beans into something that tastes great.

- 2 tablespoons avocado oil
- 1 small onion, chopped (fresh or frozen)
- 1 teaspoon garlic, minced (fresh or from a jar)
- ½ teaspoon salt
- 1 ½ teaspoons ground cumin
- 2 teaspoons chili powder
- 1 teaspoon dried oregano
- 1 can (15 oz) black beans, drained
- ½ cup water

Step 1. Heat oil in a medium saucepan and sauté onion over medium-high heat for 5 minutes.

Step 2. Add garlic and spices and cook, stirring 1 minute more.

Step 3. Add black beans and water.

Step 4. Bring to a simmer. Simmer for about 5 minutes.

Step 5. Using a potato masher, mash some of the beans in the pan to your desired texture.

Yield: 8 servings

Easy Chilaquiles

Chilaquiles make a hearty and savory breakfast that uses up leftovers. Stale tortillas are fried, then covered in sauce and toppings. Skipping a step and using corn tortilla chips saves time and is just as tasty.

- 1 bottle (19 oz) red or green enchilada sauce
- 16 ounces tortilla chips
- Salt and pepper to taste
- ½ cup cheddar cheese, shredded
- ½ cup shredded chicken
- ¼ cup black beans
- Hot sauce (optional)
- Guacamole (optional)
- 6 eggs, fried or scrambled

Step 1. Pour enchilada sauce in a wide skillet and cook over medium-high heat. Bring to a boil and allow to boil for about 3 minutes.

Step 2. Add tortilla chips, a handful at a time, folding gently to coat every chip before adding more.

Step 3. Repeat until all chips have been added and evenly coated, about 3 minutes.

Step 4. Season with salt and pepper and gently stir.

Step 5. Top with layers of cheese, chicken, beans, and hot sauce and guacamole if desired.

Step 6. Remove from heat and serve. Top each serving with a helping of eggs.

Yield: 6 servings

Legume Soaking and Cooking Instructions

There is a natural enzyme called phytase present in varying amounts inside of legumes, grains, seeds, and nuts. When this enzyme is activated, it leads to the release of healthy nutrients in the seed or grain and makes them more digestible. You must pretreat them in one of three ways, soaking, souring, or sprouting them[277] before eating if you want to activate phytase and release nutrients. For most home cooks, soaking is the easiest option.

How to soak and cook dried legumes:

Step 1. Place the dried legumes in a colander and rinse them thoroughly under cold running water to remove any dirt or debris. Transfer the rinsed legumes to a large bowl.

Step 2. Add 3–4 times the amount of water as legumes (e.g., 1 cup of legumes = 3–4 cups of water).

Optional: Add 1–2 tablespoons of an acidic medium, like lemon juice or apple cider vinegar, to the soaking water to further reduce phytic acid.

Step 3. Soak for 8–12 hours or overnight. For quicker results, use hot water and soak for 4–6 hours.

Step 4. After soaking, drain the legumes using a colander. Rinse the legumes well under cold running water to remove any residual phytic acid.

Step 5. Place the soaked and rinsed legumes in a pot and cover them with fresh water (about 2–3 times as much water as legumes).

Step 6. Bring the water to a boil over medium-high heat.

Step 7. Once boiling, reduce the heat to low, cover the pot, and simmer until tender. Cooking times vary by type:

    Beans: 45 minutes to 2 hours

    Lentils: 20–30 minutes

    Chickpeas: 1–1.5 hours

Step 8. Skim off any foam that forms on the surface during cooking.

Optional: Add salt, garlic, bay leaves, or herbs during the last 15–30 minutes of cooking. (Adding salt too early can toughen the legumes.)

Step 9. Once cooked, drain the legumes and let them cool.

Step 10. Store in an airtight container in the refrigerator for up to 5 days or freeze for longer storage.

By following these steps, you can reduce the phytate content in legumes, making them easier to digest and improving nutrient absorption.

SUMMER/FIRE RECIPES

Melon Refresher

This is a great way to use older melon for a refreshing, cooling, nourishing drink.

- 3 cups cut melon (e.g., watermelon, cantaloupe, honeydew)
- 1 cup of water
- 2 limes, juiced (4 tablespoons)

Step 1. Place cut up melon, water, and lime juice in a high-speed blender.

Step 2. Blend until smooth and enjoy.

Yield: 2–3 servings

Tomato Cucumber Bruschetta

This is a quick and easy dish to use summer's bounty. As a bonus, it feeds cells antioxidants, hydrates cells, and delivers plant medicine for the heart and immune system through the garlic, basil, and olive oil.

- 3 cups chopped tomatoes
- 1 cup chopped cucumbers
- 1 clove garlic, minced

- ¼ cup chopped fresh basil
- 2 tablespoons olive oil
- 2 tablespoons balsamic vinegar
- ½ teaspoon salt
- ¼ cup crumbled feta cheese
- Crusty bread or crackers

Step 1. In a bowl combine chopped vegetables, minced garlic, and chopped basil.

Step 2. Add olive oil, balsamic vinegar, and salt.

Step 3. Pour the feta cheese over top and mix well.

Step 4. Serve over crusty bread or with crackers.

Yield: 4–6 servings

HARVEST/EARTH RECIPES

Well Bowl Formula

This formula is a way to build a delicious, cell-healthy meal using whatever you have in your cupboards and fridge. Customize the formula with variations that work for you.

Bowl:

- 2 cups vegetables, chopped. Choose at least 3-4 types from:
  - (Raw) cucumbers, bean sprouts, shredded carrot, beets, summer squash, spinach, tomatoes, avocados, mushrooms
  - (Cooked) green beans, snap peas, sweet potatoes, winter squash, broccoli (steam beforehand), asparagus, spinach (cook briefly)
- 4 cups cooked grain (white rice, brown rice, quinoa, etc.)
- 1 tablespoon avocado oil
- 1 sauce (see recipes below for options)
- 2 cups protein (sliced beef, chicken, pork, tofu, or 4 eggs)

Sauces and Toppings:

Japanese

Sauce:
1 tablespoon soy
sauce
1 clove garlic, minced,
or 1 teaspoon pre-
minced garlic
1 teaspoon rice wine
vinegar
2 drops sriracha
sauce
Toppings:
Pickled ginger
Japanese
mayonnaise

Mexican

Sauce:
1 tablespoon pre-
made salsa
1 teaspoon cumin
½ teaspoon oregano
1 lime, juiced (2
tablespoons)
½ teaspoon salt
Toppings:
Shredded cheese
Avocado

Italian

Sauce:
2 tablespoons lemon
juice
1 tablespoon olive oil
½ teaspoon oregano
1 clove garlic, minced,
or 1 teaspoon pre-
minced garlic
1 dash black pepper
Toppings:
Parmesan cheese
Pickled peppers

Step 1. Choose a flavor profile you're in the mood for.

Step 2. Prepare the sauce and toppings for the chosen flavor profile. Mix the sauce ingredients together; set sauce and toppings aside.

Step 3. Choose 3–4 vegetables from the ingredient list; feel free to use other vegetables you have available. Plan to use a total of 2 cups of vegetables.

Step 4. Prepare 4 cups of cooked grain as directed on the package.

Step 5. Prepare the vegetables (chopping, peeling, spiralizing, etc.) as needed.

Step 6. Heat a large, wide pan or wok over medium-high heat. Add avocado oil and heat until it shimmers.

Step 7. Add vegetables that need to be cooked to the pan, starting with the vegetables that take the longest time to cook. Stir as you add to prevent burning. Continue until vegetables are cooked through.

Step 8. Heat and oil another pan and prepare your protein of choice.

Step 9. Place a portion of grain in a large bowl or on a plate. Arrange the cooked and raw vegetables and protein over the grain.

Add sauce and toppings.

Yield: 4–6 servings

Oven-Roasted Root Vegetables

Carrots, beets, and garlic add antioxidants and vitamins to traditional roasted potatoes. Vitamin A in the carrots, potassium and vitamin C in the beets, and immune-boosting allicin in the garlic.

- 3 medium potatoes (2 ½ cups), cut into bite-size chunks
- 3 medium carrots (1 ½ cups), cut into bite-size chunks
- 3 medium beets (2 ½ cups), cut into bite-size chunks
- 1 yellow onion, cut into bite-size chunks
- 5 cloves garlic, sliced
- 3 tablespoons avocado oil
- 1 teaspoon chili powder
- 1 teaspoon oregano
- 1 teaspoon kosher salt

Step 1. Preheat the oven to 425°F.

Step 2. Wash and cut the potatoes, carrots, beets, and onion. Place in a large bowl.

Step 3. Add the sliced garlic, oil, and spices.

Step 4. Toss all ingredients together. Spread out on a baking sheet.

Step 5. Cook for 30–40 minutes or until tender.

Yield: 6 servings

Cell Well Granola

It is better to eat lighter complex carbohydrates and easy-to-digest fats in the morning. This granola is the perfect blend of healthy carbs and fats and is a great way to feed your cells and generate energy for the rest of the day.

- 2 cups raw almonds
- ½ cup raw walnuts
- ½ cup raw pecans
- ½ cup raw pumpkin seeds
- ½ cup raw sunflower seeds
- ½ cup raisins (optional: additional 1 cup to mix in at end)
- 1 tablespoon vanilla extract
- ½ teaspoon cinnamon
- ½ teaspoon salt
- ¼ cup flaxseeds
- 2 tablespoons hemp seed
- 1 cup rolled oats
- ¼ cup shredded, unsweetened coconut

Step 1. Place nuts and seeds in a large bowl. Cover with water and soak for 12 hours or overnight.

Step 2. Place ½ cup raisins in a small bowl with 1 cup of water. Soak for 12 hours or overnight.

Step 3. Place soaked raisins along with their soaking water in a food processor. Puree until smooth.

Step 4. Drain and rinse nuts and seeds and discard soaking water.

Step 5. Add drained nuts and seeds to raisin puree in the food processor and pulse until coarsely chopped. (You may have to do this in two batches—if so, use half of the raisin puree in each batch).

Step 6. Add vanilla, cinnamon, salt, hemp seed, flaxseeds, and oats and pulse until mixed.

Step 7. Spread onto solid dehydrator sheets or onto a 13 x 18-inch baking sheet. Dehydrate for 12–24 hours in a dehydrator or 6–8 hours in a 175°F oven until dry all the way through.

Step 8. Place in a large bowl and add the coconut and the remaining 1 cup raisins (if desired). Mix and break granola pieces up to desired size.

Step 9. Store in a large container or ziplock bag in the fridge.

Yield: 12 cups granola

Chicken Tikka Masala

Spices are a tasty way to add nutritional value to every meal. In this very tasty dish, your cells will gain antioxidants from the tomatoes, anti-inflammatory benefits from the ginger, chili powder, and turmeric, and an immune boost from the garlic.

- 1 cup basmati rice
- 1 ½ tablespoons avocado oil
- 1 ½ pounds boneless, skinless chicken breasts, cut into 1-inch chunks
- Kosher salt and freshly ground black pepper to taste
- ½ medium sweet onion, diced
- 3 tablespoons tomato paste
- 3 cloves garlic, minced, or 3 teaspoons pre-minced garlic
- 1 tablespoon freshly grated ginger
- 1 ½ teaspoons garam masala
- 1 ½ teaspoons chili powder
- 1 ½ teaspoons ground turmeric
- 1 can (15 oz) tomato sauce
- 1 cup chicken stock

- ½ cup heavy cream
- 2 tablespoons chopped fresh cilantro (optional)

Step 1. Cook rice according to package instructions; set aside.

Step 2. Heat oil in a large stockpot over medium heat.

Step 3. Season chicken with salt and pepper.

Step 4. Add chicken and onion to the stockpot and cook until golden, about 4–5 minutes.

Step 5. Stir in tomato paste, garlic, ginger, garam masala, chili powder, and turmeric until fragrant, about 1 minute.

Step 6. Stir in tomato sauce and chicken stock. Season with salt and pepper to taste.

Step 7. Bring to a boil. Reduce heat and simmer, stirring occasionally, until liquid is reduced and slightly thickened, about 10 minutes.

Step 8. Stir in heavy cream until heated through, about 1 minute.

Step 9. Serve immediately with rice. Garnish with cilantro, if desired.

Yield: 6–8 servings

Dr. Michelle's Adaptogenic Golden Milk

This drink, with its anti-inflammatory turmeric and ginger, will warm and soothe your cells and you.

- 2 cups coconut, oat, or almond milk
- 1 teaspoon ground turmeric
- ¼ teaspoon ground ginger
- 1 teaspoon vanilla extract

- ¼ teaspoon cinnamon
- 1 pinch black pepper
- Honey to taste

Step 1. In a blender, combine all ingredients. Blend together until smooth.

Step 2. Warm gently on the stove until desired temperature is reached.

Yield: 1 serving

Savory Crockpot Lentil Stew

This recipe comes together in 15 minutes, and is ready to eat in the evening. The lentils are full of complex carbohydrates for energy, the tomatoes deliver vitamin C and antioxidants, and the spices bring your cells immune-boosting and anti-inflammatory benefits.

- 1 tablespoon avocado oil
- ½ onion, diced
- 2 carrots, diced
- 2 cloves garlic, minced, or 2 teaspoons pre-minced garlic
- 1 bay leaf
- 2 teaspoons cumin
- 1 teaspoon paprika
- 1 teaspoon oregano
- 1 teaspoon sea salt
- ½ teaspoon pepper
- 1 ¼ cups dried brown lentils, rinsed
- 1 can (14.5 oz) white beans
- 1 can (14.5 oz) diced tomatoes
- 1 can (8 oz) tomato sauce
- 3 cups vegetable broth
- ½ cup spinach, torn into bite-sized pieces

Step 1. In a large pot, heat oil and sauté the onion, carrots, and garlic until tender. Add spices and cook for 2 more minutes.

Step 2. Stir in lentils, white beans, tomatoes, tomato sauce, and vegetable broth. Bring to a boil. Reduce heat and simmer on the stovetop for about an hour, or put into a slow cooker and cook on low for 6–8 hours.

Step 3. When ready to serve, add spinach and salt and pepper to taste.

Step 4. Serve the stew hot with your favorite toppings.

Yield: 6–8 servings

FALL/AIR RECIPES

Cellular Oxygen Smoothie

This smoothie brings your cells vitamin C and other antioxidants, as well as important minerals and fiber, that support digestion and oxygen utilization in your body.

- 1 cup fresh spinach
- ½ cup frozen blueberries
- ½ banana
- 1 small beet, cut into chunks
- ½ banana
- 1 cup coconut water or almond milk
- A squeeze of lemon juice
- 1 teaspoon honey (optional)
- 1 tablet calcium lactate to counteract the oxalates in the greens (optional)

Step 1. Wash the spinach and beet.

Step 2. Combine all ingredients in a blender and blend until smooth. Taste and add more honey if needed.

Yield: 1 serving

Cold-Busting Ginger-ade

This has been touted as "the best thing to fight a cold since Mom's chicken soup"—and that claim has been proven true time and time again. With lemon juice for vitamin C, ginger to fight inflammation, cayenne to rev up the body's healing systems, and honey to soothe, this is the first thing I make when anyone is sick in my home.

- 1 quart water
- 1 tablespoon grated ginger
- 1 dash cayenne
- 2 tablespoons lemon juice
- ¼ cup honey

Step 1. Bring the water to a boil and add the ginger and cayenne.

Step 2. Simmer, covered, for 15 minutes.

Step 3. Strain out all solids and add the lemon juice and honey to taste.

Step 4. Drink 1–2 cups every few hours until feeling better.

Yield: 3–4 servings

Everyone's Favorite Spinach Salad

This salad recipe has graced dinner tables in my family for years. The spinach provides folate, crucial for DNA synthesis and repair, the mushrooms bring B vitamins for energy production, the boiled eggs and cheese provide amino acids for cell growth, and the olive oil protects the heart and reduces inflammation. Make sure to add the dressing; it is the star of the salad.

- 6 cups torn spinach or dark greens
- ½ cup mushrooms, cut up
- 4 green onions, diced
- 1 cup shredded mozzarella cheese

- 2 boiled eggs, chopped
- 1 recipe Healthy Poppy Seed Dressing (recipe below)

Step 1. Wash the salad greens thoroughly. Pat dry with a clean kitchen towel or dry with salad spinner. Tear the greens into bite-sized pieces if they are large.

Step 2. Place the spinach or dark salad greens in a large salad bowl.

Step 3. Add the chopped mushrooms and green onions to the bowl.

Step 4. Top with the chopped boiled eggs. Sprinkle on cheese.

Step 5. Mix as desired. Serve with Healthy Poppy Seed Dressing.

Yield: 6–8 servings

Healthy Poppy Seed Dressing

- ½ cup raw honey
- ½ cup cider vinegar
- 1 cup extra virgin olive oil
- 1 tablespoon yellow mustard
- 1 teaspoon salt
- 1 small red onion, quartered
- 1 tablespoon poppy seeds

Step 1. Blend all ingredients except the poppy seeds in a blender.

Step 2. Add poppy seeds and pulse a couple of times.

Step 3. Keep refrigerated until use.

Yield 2 ¼ cups dressing

Creamy Cell Well Hummus

Hummus is great eaten with other healthy plants like carrot and celery sticks because the chickpeas help with energy production, the garlic boosts the immune system, the tahini supports your heart health, and the lemon juice rounds out this nutrition powerhouse with vitamin C.

- 1 can (15 oz) chickpeas, rinsed and drained
- 1 clove garlic, roughly chopped
- ½ teaspoon baking soda
- 1 ½–2 lemons, juiced (¼ cup lemon juice)
- ½ teaspoon salt
- ½ cup tahini
- 2–4 tablespoons ice water
- ½ teaspoon ground cumin
- 1 tablespoon olive oil
- Paprika (optional)

Step 1. Place the chickpeas and clove of garlic in a saucepan with the baking soda.

Step 2. Cover with several inches of water and boil for 10 minutes.

Step 3. In a fine-mesh strainer, drain the chickpeas and garlic. Set aside.

Step 4. In a food processor, combine the lemon juice and salt. Process for 30 seconds.

Step 5. Add tahini to the food processor and blend until the mixture is thick and creamy, scraping down the sides as necessary.

Step 6. While food processor is running, drizzle in ice water. Scrape down the sides, and blend until the mixture is ultra-smooth. Add the cumin and the drained chickpeas and garlic.

Step 7. Blend until the mixture is very smooth, about 2 minutes.

Step 8. Add more ice water by the tablespoon if necessary to achieve a creamy texture. Taste and adjust as necessary.

Step 9. Spoon the hummus into a serving bowl or platter. Use a spoon to create swirling depressions on top. Pour olive oil into the depressions. Sprinkle with paprika to garnish.

Yield: 4 servings

Miso Glazed Salmon

Miso brings umami flavor which makes you want more of whatever you're eating. As a bonus, the salmon is full of healthy fats for better cell signaling, and the miso contains gut-healthy probiotics.

- ¼ cup red or white miso
- ⅓ cup sake or white wine
- 1 tablespoon soy sauce
- 2 tablespoons avocado oil
- 2 tablespoon honey
- 4 skinless salmon filets, at least 1 inch thick (5–6 oz each)

Step 1. In a large bowl whisk together miso, sake, soy sauce, oil, and honey.

Step 2. Rub mixture over every surface of salmon filets.

Step 3. Transfer to a plastic ziplock bag or sealable container. Marinate for about 30 minutes.

Step 4. Preheat broiler to high.

Step 5. Cover a sheet pan with parchment. Use a spoon to remove excess marinade off salmon and place the filets on the pan.

Step 6. Broil until top surface is slightly blackened and the salmon is warm in the center, about 5 minutes.

Step 7. Serve immediately.

Yield: 4 servings

Cell Well No-Bake Cookies

These cookies are filled with cell-healthy nutrients, and kids and adults alike love them. Easy to throw together, they bring your cells heart-healthy fats, fiber-filled grains, and antioxidant- and mineral-rich cocoa powder. Yum!

- 4 cups rolled oats
- ½ cup almond butter or tahini
- ½ cup coconut oil
- 1 tablespoon vanilla
- 6 tablespoons cocoa powder
- ¾ cup honey
- ½ teaspoon salt
- 2 tablespoons chia seeds

Step 1. In a large bowl, mix all wet ingredients together.

Step 2. Add dry ingredients to the same bowl. Mix well.

Step 3. By the spoonful, scoop and drop onto a baking sheet.

Step 4. Place in the freezer until hard.

Step 5. Store in the fridge.

Yield: 12–16 cookies

WINTER/WATER RECIPES

No-Bake Fruit Crumble

The fresh fruit in this crumble has more nutrient value, vitamins, minerals, and enzymes than the same fruit when it's cooked. Your family will be glad you found this recipe, and you will, too. You can make it in a quick ten minutes!

- 2 cups fresh fruit (cut-up apples, pears, berries, or a combination)
- 1 cup rolled oats
- ¼ cup coconut oil
- 1 teaspoon cinnamon
- ½ cup chopped nuts
- ½ cup golden raisins
- 4 teaspoons honey
- ½ teaspoon salt

Step 1. Place cut-up fruit in a medium-sized serving bowl.

Step 2. In a separate bowl, combine all other ingredients and mix well to make a crumble.

Step 3. Top the cut-up fruit with the crumble mixture.

Step 4. Serve with sweetened yogurt, cream, or coconut cream if desired.

Yield: 4–6 servings

Healthy Kidney Black Bean Soup

This is the meal you want to make for a crowd, and it's especially nice on a cold winter day. Full of vitamins and minerals from the vegetables and beans, eating a bowl is sure to turn your appestat to "full."

- 1 tablespoon avocado oil
- 1 large yellow onion, chopped
- 1 large carrot, chopped
- 1 red bell pepper, stemmed, seeded, and chopped
- 4 cloves garlic, minced, or 4 teaspoons pre-minced garlic
- 4 cans (15 oz each) black beans, rinsed and drained
- 1 quart vegetable broth
- 1 tablespoon ground cumin
- ½ teaspoon oregano
- 1 bay leaf
- Salt and black pepper to taste
- ½ lime, juiced (1 tablespoon)
- ¼ cup chopped cilantro
- 1 avocado, sliced

Step 1. In a large pot, heat oil over medium high heat.

Step 2. Add the onion, carrot, and red pepper. Cook until vegetables are tender, about 5 minutes.

Step 3. Add garlic and cook for another 2 minutes.

Step 4. Stir in the black beans, vegetable broth, cumin, oregano, bay leaf, salt, and pepper. Turn the heat to low and let simmer for 25 minutes.

Step 5. Remove the bay leaf.

Step 6. Stir in the cilantro and fresh lime juice. Top with avocado and enjoy!

Yield: 8 servings

Cell Well Miso Soup

After I found out miso soup was a great source of electrolytes, I wanted to make it at home, so I learned how to make broth—and you can, too! Find these ingredients online or at an Asian market near you.

- 6 cups water
- 1 piece dried kombu
- 1 package bonito flakes
- 2 tablespoons dried wakame
- ¼ cup miso (white miso is the mildest)
- 1 tablespoon sliced green onion
- 1 cup extra firm tofu, cut into small cubes

Step 1. In a large pot, bring water to a boil. Turn off the heat.

Step 2. Add the kombu and bonito flakes and let sit, without heating, for 15 min.

Step 3. Strain out all flakes and seaweed and return broth to the pot.

Step 4. Add tofu and green onions. Crumble dried wakame into broth.

Step 5. Remove ½ cup of broth and gently stir miso into the removed broth until mixed. Add miso and broth back to the pot. Do not boil.

Yield: 4 servings

APPENDIX 2

Well Home Cleaning Products

Some of the most toxic chemicals in your life are found in the products you use to clean your home. When you spray and wipe with these things, you inhale and touch chemicals you would never put in your body otherwise. The good news is this is one of the easiest areas to "clean up." Many effective household cleaners can be made from ingredients you already have in your kitchen.

Everything in this appendix can also be found at www.resources .livingwellbook.com.

Kitchen and Bath All-Purpose Cleaner

- ½ cup white vinegar
- 2 tablespoons baking soda
- 3 cups water
- 5 drops essential oil (tea tree, eucalyptus, or citrus)

Step 1. Mix all ingredients in a full-sized spray bottle. Shake well.

Step 2. Spray on kitchen and bath surfaces and wipe off with a clean cloth.

Yield: 4 cups

Mirror Cleaner

· ·

- ½ cup water
- ½ cup vinegar

Step 1. Mix together in a spray bottle.

Step 2. Spray on the mirror and wipe off. Use a microfiber cloth for no streaks or cloth fibers left behind.

Yield: 1 cup

Toilet Cleaner

· ·

- ½ cup vinegar
- 1 teaspoon baking soda

Step 1. Put vinegar into a spray bottle and spray onto the surface.

Step 2. Scrub with a toilet brush. Sprinkle baking soda on top of vinegar for more scrubbing power.

Yield: ½ cup

APPENDIX 3

Well Body Products

Even people who work hard to keep their food "clean" often give little thought to the products they use on their face or body. Here is a sampling of recipes you can use to create your own clean, simple, toxin-free beauty products at home.

Everything in this appendix can also be found at www.resources .livingwellbook.com.

Simple Face Moisturizer

- ½ cup shea butter
- 2 tablespoons organic coconut oil
- 2 tablespoons organic extra virgin olive oil
- 20 drops frankincense, lavender, or rose essential oil (optional)

Step 1. Add all the ingredients to a glass mason jar or small glass bowl.

Step 2. Place the bowl or jar into a pan of simmering water, making sure no water gets into the bowl or jar. Stir until melted.

Step 3. Carefully remove the bowl or jar from the water and pour into a smaller glass jar. Cool and store at room temperature.

Step 4. Use a pea-sized amount every day to moisturize your face.

Yield: ¾ cup (enough for 6 months of use)

Nonallergenic Face Powder

- ¼ cup arrowroot powder

As needed to match your complexion:

- Unsweetened cocoa powder
- Cinnamon
- Ginger
- Bentonite clay

Step 1. Put the arrowroot in a glass bowl. This will be your base.

Step 2. Add the other ingredients a little at a time until you reach the shade that matches your complexion. Test by placing the mixture on your forearm. Continue to adjust as needed.

Step 3. Store your face powder in a small container and use a dry sponge or brush to apply.

Yield: ⅓ cup

APPENDIX 4

Seasonal Body and Lifestyle Recommendations

As you've learned, Living Well isn't just about what you eat or put on your skin, it's also very much about how you use your body, remove waste, and power the energy in your cells. This section contains all the body and lifestyle recommendations found in *Living Well with Dr. Michelle.*

Everything in this appendix can also be found at www.resources .livingwellbook.com.

Seasonal Body and Lifestyle Recommendations Index

Dry Brushing Instructions

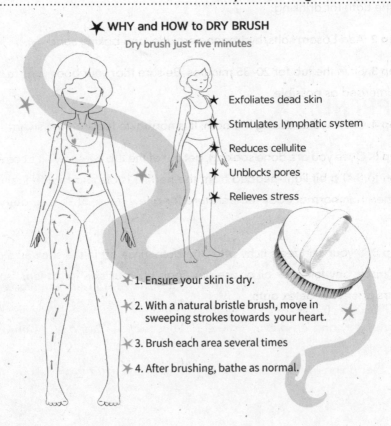

✴ WHY and HOW to DRY BRUSH

Dry brush just five minutes

- ✴ Exfoliates dead skin
- ✴ Stimulates lymphatic system
- ✴ Reduces cellulite
- ✴ Unblocks pores
- ✴ Relieves stress

✴ 1. Ensure your skin is dry.

✴ 2. With a natural bristle brush, move in sweeping strokes towards your heart.

✴ 3. Brush each area several times

✴ 4. After brushing, bathe as normal.

Detox Bath Instructions

This detox bath is full of beneficial ingredients, which your skin absorbs as you soak and relax. Epsom salts detox, reduce inflammation, lower blood pressure, promote healthy circulation, and help with relaxation and sleep. Meanwhile, hydrogen peroxide increases oxygenation of the blood, and baking soda supports digestion issues and combats sore throat (including strep throat).

- 2 cups Epsom salts
- 1 cup hydrogen peroxide
- 1 cup baking soda

Step 1. Fill your bath with very hot water. Set a glass of water to the side of the bath for drinking.

Step 2. Add Epsom salts, hydrogen peroxide, and baking soda.

Step 3. Sit in the tub for 20-35 minutes. Be sure that your body is as fully submerged as possible.

Step 4. Drink water during the bath. It is normal to feel hot and sweat.

Step 5. Once you are done soaking, get out of the tub carefully—it's common to feel a bit light-headed from the heat. It is also normal to feel a higher than normal body temperature for a few hours after your detox bath.

Step 6. If your skin feels itchy after the bath, rinse off in the shower. *Do not* apply any lotion or oil or use any soap on your skin for at least six hours after your detox bath.

Well Lung Breathing Exercises

Well Lung Breathing Exercises

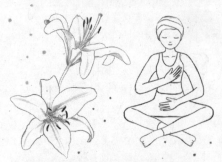

Deep Breathing (Diaphragmatic Breathing)

Inhale deeply through your nose,
expanding your diaphragm,
then exhale slowly through your
mouth.
Focus on the breath filling your lungs.

*Benefits: Removes phlegm in the throat
and improves oxygenation.*

Alternate Nostril Breathing (Nadi Shodhana)

Inhale through one nostril, close it with
your thumb, and exhale through the
other nostril. Repeat on the other side.

*Benefits: Balances energy levels and helps
release stress and anxiety.*

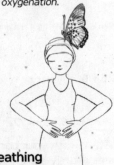

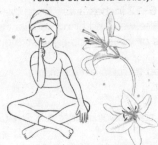

Belly Breathing (Ujjayi)

Breathe deeply, filling your belly, and exhale slowly.
Constrict the back of your throat slightly
to create a soft hissing sound during both
inhales and exhales.

*Benefits: Helps in relaxation, lowering heart rate,
and reducing blood pressure.*

Wall Angel Instructions

Wall Angel

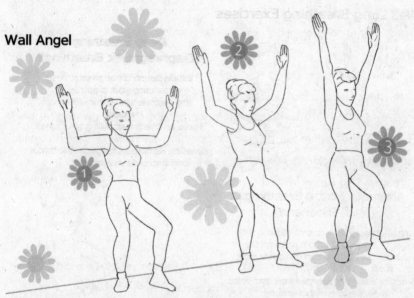

1. Stand with your back against the wall, feet 6–12 inches away from the wall, knees slightly bent. Flatten your back against the wall and bring your arms up at 90 degrees, with your elbows and the backs of your hands against the wall.

2. Slowly straighten your arms above your head to form a Y position, maintaining contact with the wall until straight.

3. Bring your arms back to a 90 degree angle, then back up into a Y Position.

Try 3 sets of 10, which you can space throughout the day to help keep you moving and mobile.

Living Well Yoga Instructions and Season/Element Poses

Illustrations for all poses can be found at www.resources.livingwellbook.com.

Choosing Poses: Using the Cell Well Seasonal yoga poses list as a guide, select poses that correspond with the Season or Element you're focusing on. For example, for winter, you might choose grounding and warming poses, while for the summer, cooling and heart-opening poses might be more appropriate.

Warm-Up: Begin with a gentle warm-up, including light stretching and breathing exercises (page 334) to prepare your body.

Holding Poses

- **Beginner Level:** Hold each pose for fifteen to thirty seconds.
- **Intermediate Level:** Hold each pose for thirty to sixty seconds.
- **Advanced Level:** Hold each pose for one to two minutes or longer.

Frequency

Perform each pose two to three times in a session to fully experience its benefits. **Aim for 3–4 sessions per week.**

Yoga Routines for Each Season/Element
Spring/Plants
Poses: Cow Pose, Skull Shining Breath, Half Lord of the Fishes, Boat Pose

Complementary Practices: Focus on cleansing and a light diet rich in fresh, seasonal produce.

Summer/Fire
Poses: Twisted Roots, Bananasana, One-Legged Downward Dog, Revolved Child's Pose, Sphinx Pose, Supported Backbend

Complementary Practices: Emphasize cooling practices including hydration and deep breathing in through the mouth and out through the nose.

Harvest/Earth

Poses: Bridge Pose, Cobra Pose, High Lunge, Tree Pose, Chair Pose, Boat Pose, Camel Pose, Sun Salutations

Complementary Practices: Focus on grounding and stability. Practice mindfulness meditation.

Fall/Air

Poses: Seated Pranayama, Pec Stretch at Wall, Cat Pulling Its Tail, Supported Bridge Pose, Open Wing, Supine Butterfly Pose

Complementary Practices: Focus on movement, change, and balance. Practice meditation focused on breathing and letting go of any stress or tension.

Winter/Water

Poses: Child's Pose, Three-Legged Downward Dog, Low Lunge, Upward-Facing Dog, Plank Pose, Downward-Facing Dog, Garland Pose, Warrior Pose 2, Butterfly Pose

Complementary Practices: Emphasize warmth and fluidity. Practice gentle, flowing movements and include restorative yoga in your sessions.

Additional Tips

Listen to your body. Always pay attention to how your body feels during each pose. Modify poses as needed to avoid strain.

Be consistent. Regular practice is key to experiencing the benefits of yoga. Aim for consistency rather than perfection.

Pay attention to hydration and nutrition. Maintain proper hydration and consume a balanced diet that supports your yoga practice and overall health.

By following these guidelines, you can create a balanced and effective Seasonal/Elemental yoga practice that supports your physical, mental, and emotional well-being.

Well Week Exercise Guide

Weekly Exercise Routine

Monday	Tuesday	Wednesday	Thursday	Friday	Saturday	Sunday
Cardio	**Strength**	**Cardio**	**Strength**	**Cardio**	**Cardio**	**Cardio**
15-min walk after lunch and dinner	1-2 sets of 8 each Bodyweight squat Push-up Bird dog T-spine rotation Side lunge	15-min walk after lunch and dinner	1-2 sets of 8 each Bodyweight squat Push-up Bird dog T-spine rotation Side lunge	15-min walk after lunch and dinner	15-min walk after lunch and dinner	15-min walk after lunch and dinner
Flexibility	**Flexibility**	**Flexibility**	**Flexibility**	**Flexibility**	**Flexibility**	**Flexibility**
Spend 5 mins stretching Child's Pose Leg Crossover Stretch Spinal Twist	Spend 5 mins stretching Child's Pose Leg Crossover Stretch Spinal Twist	Spend 5 mins stretching Child's Pose Leg Crossover stretch Spinal Twist	Spend 5 mins stretching Child's Pose Leg Crossover Stretch Spinal Twist	Spend 5 mins stretching Child's Pose Leg Crossover Stretch Spinal Twist	Spend 5 mins stretching Child's Pose Leg Crossover Stretch Spinal Twist	Spend 5 mins stretching Child's Pose Leg Crossover Stretch Spinal Twist

Bird Dog

Bodyweight Squat

Child's Pose

Leg Crossover Stretch

Spinal Twist

Side Lunge

Living Well Acupressure Protocol

Acupressure is a traditional Chinese medicine technique that involves applying pressure to specific points on the body to promote relaxation, reduce stress, and enhance overall well-being. Below is a protocol for using acupressure points to support wellness.

Preparation

1. **Choose a Quiet Space:** Find a quiet, comfortable place where you won't be disturbed.

2. **Relax and Breathe:** Take a few deep breaths before starting.

3. **Warm Up:** Rub your hands together to create warmth and energy.

Key Acupressure Points for Wellness

(Use the appropriate points for each Season/Element, as illustrated below.)

General Protocol

1. **Pressure and Duration:** Apply firm but comfortable pressure. Spend 1–2 minutes on each point, massaging in a circular motion.
2. **Frequency:** Practice acupressure 2–3 times a day for general wellness. For specific issues, increase the frequency.

Complementary Practices

- **Hydration:** Drink plenty of water before and after the session to help flush out toxins.
- **Deep Breathing:** Incorporate deep breathing exercises into the acupressure session to enhance relaxation.

Safety Tips

- **Avoid Injured Areas:** Do not apply pressure to areas with cuts, bruises, or other injuries.
- **Pregnancy:** Consult with a health-care provider before using acupressure during pregnancy, as some points may induce labor.
- **Medical Conditions:** If you have a serious health condition, consult with a health-care professional before starting acupressure.

Spring/Plants Points: Liver 3, Gallbladder 34

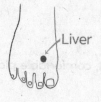
Liver

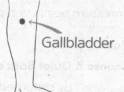
Gallbladder

Summer/Fire Points: Heart 7 and 9, Pericardium 7 and 9, Small Intestine 3 and 8

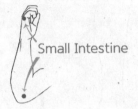

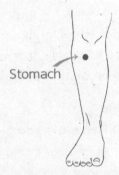

Harvest/Earth Points: Spleen 6 and 9, Stomach 36

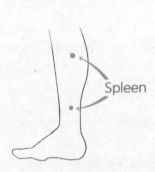

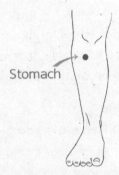

Fall/Air Points: Large Intestine 4, Lung 9

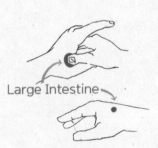

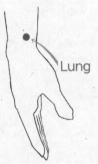

Winter/Water Points: Kidney 1, Spleen 6 and 9

Kidney

Spleen

ACKNOWLEDGMENTS

I like to joke that in a previous life I was Mother Earth's assistant. She opened my eyes to the harmony and synergy between the earth, its Seasons, and its Elements. Now, as I teach others about these natural cycles and how they can assist us in living well, it all feels very familiar.

This book has been in the making for what feels like ages. Every piece of information in this book stems from small experiences or memories shared with mentors and friends. The feel of warm, crumbly earth and the juicy bite of a tree-ripened peach bring back fond memories of gardening and preserving with my grandmother Shirley, my mother Sue, and her seven younger sisters. They were my first teachers. From there, I learned how to use foods and plants for medicine, thanks to mentors like Marjory Wildcraft, Robyn Openshaw, and Karen Urbanek. They inspired me to ask questions—inside and outside of my profession—that helped me continue to learn from pioneers who dared to step off the beaten path.

Those brave practitioners taught me that I didn't have to choose between one approach or another. I could merge my knowledge of Mother Earth with my scientific studies to create a more complete model of health care. Special thanks go to Dr. Evan Brady, Dr. Paul Jones, Dr. Judson Wall, Dr. Thomas Levy, Dr. Jerry Tennant, Dr. Matthew Hollist, Dr. Jessica Herzog, Dr. Karl Volz, and many others who helped pave the way for me.

I've self-published five books on various topics, each one a joyful and inspired experience. But this book is different. It's more than just another project; this book represents a mission. The goal of this book—and all my work with Living Well with Dr. Michelle—is to help *you* and others reclaim the ability to live well. As someone recently said to me, "We are the CEOs of our own bodies." And that's true—but no one becomes a CEO overnight. You need training, practice, and experience to step into the role. This book is your CEO training manual.

I knew I needed to reach a wider audience, and for that, I sought the exposure that a traditional publisher could offer. I was fortunate to connect with an amazing agent, Nena Oshman, who guided me through the process. She helped me shape two out-of-the-box concepts into the book you hold today and showed my publisher its potential. Glenn Yeffeth at BenBella Books took a chance on this dentist-turned-author, and together, we brought this book to life.

The publishing team was surprised to learn that I intended to write the book on my own, without a coauthor or ghostwriter (naively, I assumed that's how all books were written!). They were even more surprised to hear that I'd be doing this while running two businesses full-time. But I approached writing the same way I approach anything daunting: I created a schedule and stuck to it. Along the way, I leaned on those I trust. My partners, Dr. Lyndi Jones and Dr. Tyler Coles, along with my teams at Total Care Dental and Living Well with Dr. Michelle, shouldered much of the workload while I wrote.

Two other key people were by my side throughout this journey. My best friend, coach, and mentor, Karyn Ross, who has published numerous books, provided endless content and editorial help. She edited every word of *Living Well with Dr. Michelle*—twice!—and served as a voice of reason, clarity, and unwavering encouragement. Her input was invaluable, especially as many concepts were new to her. She helped me simplify complex scientific ideas so that everyone could understand them. This book, and the Cell Well model it introduces, wouldn't be what they are today without her guidance and editorial brilliance.

As I started writing, I quickly realized that illustrations would be crucial in bringing both the book and the model to life. I wanted visuals that were beautiful, nature-based, and a little whimsical, while still scientifically accurate. When I found a book with just the style I wanted, I took a brave step and reached out to the illustrator. To my delight, Ruth Evans, artist extraordinaire, was intrigued by the project. Ruth and her son, Finn Evans, worked within tight deadlines and delivered illustrations that far exceeded my expectations.

Finally, and most importantly, I want to thank my family. My husband, Steve, took over early-morning and late-night family duties while I wrote in my cottage. He was a patient listener when I vented about writer's block and indulged my ramblings about studies I was excited to share. Not once did he complain or roll his eyes at his "crazy" wife! My children—Jens, Brooklyn, Josh, Luke, and Liza—and my grandbabies, Mira and Cohen, stepped up and filled the gaps I would normally take care of, all without hesitation. I love you all, and I'm so glad I can help you live well, too.

NOTES

....

1. YouGov. "Americans Who Made 2024 New Year's Resolutions Say They Have Stuck to Them." Accessed May 19, 2024. https://today.yougov.com/society/articles/49045-americans-who-made-2024-new-years-resolutions-say-they-have-stuck-to-them.

2. Luther, Claudia. "Jack LaLanne Dies at 96; Spiritual Father of U.S. Fitness Movement." *Los Angeles Times*, January 23, 2011. Accessed April 13, 2024. https://www.latimes.com/local/obituaries/la-me-jack-lalanne-20110124-story.html.

3. Winston Medical Center. "Human Brain Facts." Accessed May 19, 2024. https://www.winstonmedical.org/human-brain-facts/.

4. Timmer, John. "You're a Dim Bulb, and I Mean That in the Best Possible Way." *Discover Magazine*. Accessed May 19, 2024. https://www.discovermagazine.com/mind/youre-a-dim-bulb-and-i-mean-that-in-the-best-possible-way.

5. Cleveland Clinic. "Fun Facts About Your Heart." Accessed May 19, 2024. https://health.clevelandclinic.org/fun-facts-about-your-heart.

6. Yagi, Shinya, Mitsuhisa Hirata, Yoshinori Miyachi, and Shinji Uemoto. "Liver Regeneration Hepatectomy and Partial Liver Transplantation." *International Journal of Molecular Sciences* 21, no. 21 (November 9, 2020): 8414. https://doi.org/10.3390/ijms21218414. PMID: 33182515; PMCID: PMC7665117.

7. Scientific American. "Our Bodies Replace Billions of Cells Every Day." Accessed May 19, 2024. https://www.scientificamerican.com/article/our-bodies-replace-billions-of-cells-every-day/.

8. Peterson-Kaiser Health System Tracker. "How Does Health Spending in the U.S. Compare to Other Countries?" Accessed November 3, 2024. https://www.healthsystemtracker.org/chart-collection/health-spending-u-s-compare-countries/#GDP%20per%20capita%20and%20health%20consumption%20spending%20per%20capita,%202022%20(U.S.%20dollars,%20PPP%20adjusted).

9. "U.S. Adults Spend Eight Hours Monthly Coordinating Healthcare, Find System 'Overwhelming.'" *American Academy of Physician Assistants*, May 17, 2023. Accessed April 13, 2024. https://www.aapa.org/news-central/2023/05/u-s-adults-spend-eight-hours-monthly-coordinating-healthcare-find-system-overwhelming/.

10. "Life Expectancy in the U.S. Dropped for the Second Year in a Row in 2021." *Centers for Disease Control and Prevention*. August 31, 2022. Accessed April 13, 2024. https://www.cdc.gov/nchs/pressroom/nchs_press_releases/2022/20220831.htm.

11. Dattani, Saloni, Lucas Rodés-Guirao, Hannah Ritchie, Esteban Ortiz-Ospina, and Max Roser. "Life Expectancy." *Our World in Data*. Published 2023. https://ourworldindata.org/life-expectancy.

12. World Health Organization. "GHE: Life Expectancy and Healthy Life Expectancy." Accessed November 3, 2024. https://www.who.int/data/gho/data/themes/mortality-and-global-health-estimates/ghe-life-expectancy-and-healthy-life-expectancy.

13. The Senior List. "Senior Living Industry Statistics in 2024." Accessed November 3, 2024. https://www.theseniorlist.com/senior-housing/statistics/.

14. Forbes. "Assisted Living Statistics and Facts in 2024." Forbes Health. January 11, 2024. Accessed April 13, 2024. https://www.forbes.com/health/senior-living/assisted-living-statistics/.

15. Grand View Research. "U.S. Assisted Living Facility Market Size & Share Report, 2030." Accessed April 13, 2024. https://www.grandviewresearch.com/industry-analysis/us-assisted-living-facility-market.

16. Geyer, S., and S. Eberhard. "Compression and Expansion of Morbidity—Secular Trends Among Cohorts of the Same Age." *Deutsches Arzteblatt International* 119, no. 47 (2022): 810–815. https://doi.org/10.3238/arztebl.m2022.0324.

17. Zheng, H. and P. Echave. "Are Recent Cohorts Getting Worse? Trends in US Adult Physiological Status, Mental Health, and Health Behaviors Across a Century of Birth Cohorts." *American Journal of Epidemiology* 190, no. 11 (2021): 2242–2255. https://doi.org/10.1093/aje/kwab076.

18. World Health Organization (WHO). "Obesity and Overweight." Accessed March 1, 2024. https://www.who.int/news-room/fact-sheets/detail/obesity-and-overweight.

19. Ibid. Accessed March 1, 2024

20. Perrin, J. M., L. E. Anderson, and J. Van Cleave. "The Rise in Chronic Conditions Among Infants, Children, and Youth Can Be Met with Continued Health System Innovations." *Health Affairs* 33, no. 12 (2014): 2099–2105. https://doi.org/10.1377/hlthaff.2014.0832.

21. Angelo, A. "Are Environmental Toxins Haunting Our Kids?" *Environmental Health Sciences Center*. Accessed October 13, 2022. https://environmentalhealth.ucdavis.edu/blog/children-environmental-health-month.

22. Harvard T.H. Chan School of Public Health. "Children's Health—C-CHANGE." Accessed April 13, 2024. https://www.hsph.harvard.edu/c-change/subtopics/climate-change-and-childrens-health/.

23. Lebrun-Harris, Landrine A., Ruth M. Ghandour, Michael D. Kogan, and Michelle D. Warren. "Five-Year Trends in US Children's Health and Well-being, 2016–2020." *JAMA Pediatrics* 176, no. 7 (2022): e220056. https://doi.org/10.1001/jamapediatrics.2022.0056.

24. Our World in Data. "Life Expectancy." Accessed April 13, 2024. https://ourworldindata.org/life-expectancy.

25. McNeill, Laura. "SJ Baker: The New Yorker Who Saved 90,000 Infants." *BBC*, May 17, 2020. Accessed April 13, 2024. https://www.bbc.com/future/article/20200514-sj -baker-the-new-york-woman-who-transformed-public-health.

26. Shapiro-Shapin, C. G. "Pearl Kendrick, Grace Eldering, and the Pertussis Vaccine." *Emerging Infectious Diseases* 16, no. 8 (2010): 1273–1278. https://doi.org/10.3201 /eid1608.100288.

27. Gibbon, Paul. "Jane Addams: A Hero for Our Time." *The National Endowment for the Humanities*. Accessed April 13, 2024. https://www.neh.gov/article/jane-addams -hero-our-time.

28. Klein, Christopher. "How Upton Sinclair's 'The Jungle' Led to US Food Safety Reforms." *HISTORY*. Accessed April 13, 2024. https://www.history.com/news/upton -sinclair-the-jungle-us-food-safety-reforms.

29. "Straus Family." *Britannica*. Accessed April 13, 2024. https://www.britannica.com /topic/Straus-family.

30. Garmany, Anne, Shigeki Yamada, and Andre Terzic. "Longevity Leap: Mind the Healthspan Gap." *NPJ Regenerative Medicine* 6, no. 1 (September 23, 2021): 57. https://doi.org/10.1038/s41536-021-00169-5.

31. "History of the Cell: Discovering the Cell." *National Geographic Society*. Accessed April 13, 2024. https://education.nationalgeographic.org/resource/history-cell-discovering-cell/.

32. Wikipedia. (n.d.). Robert Hooke. Wikipedia. Retrieved April 13, 2024, from https:// en.wikipedia.org/wiki/Robert_Hooke.

33. MedlinePlus. "What Is a Cell?" *MedlinePlus Genetics*. U.S. National Library of Medicine. Accessed August 23, 2024. https://medlineplus.gov/genetics/understanding /basics/cell/.

34. Kelly, K., M. Posternak, and J.E. Alpert. "Toward Achieving Optimal Response: Understanding and Managing Antidepressant Side Effects." *Dialogues in Clinical Neuroscience* 10, no. 4 (2008): 409–18. https://doi.org/10.31887/DCNS.2008.10 .4/kkelly. PMID: 19170398; PMCID: PMC3181894.

35. Geier, David and Mark Geier. "Dental Amalgam Fillings and Mercury Vapor Safety Limits in American Adults." *Human & Experimental Toxicology* 41 (2022): 096032712211063. https://doi.org/10.1177/09603271221106341.

36. Nix, Elizabeth. "Where Did the Phrase 'Mad as a Hatter' Come From?" December 3, 2015. Accessed April 15, 2024. https://www.history.com/news/where-did-the-phrase -mad-as-a-hatter-come-from.

37. U.S. Food and Drug Administration. "Dental Amalgam Fillings." *FDA*. Last modified August 7, 2023. https://www.fda.gov/medical-devices/dental-devices/dental -amalgam-fillings.

38. Carocci, Alessia, Nicola Rovito, Maria Stefania Sinicropi, and Genchi Genchi. "Mercury Toxicity and Neurodegenerative Effects." *Reviews of Environmental Contamination and Toxicology* (December 31, 2013): 1–18. https://doi.org/10.1007/978-3-319 -03777-6_1.

39. Rodríguez-Viso, Paula, Alba Domene, Daniel Vélez, Victor Devesa, Victor Monedero, and Maria Zúñiga. "Mercury Toxic Effects on the Intestinal Mucosa Assayed on a

Bicameral In Vitro Model: Possible Role of Inflammatory Response and Oxidative Stress." *Food and Chemical Toxicology* 166 (August 2022): 113224. https://doi.org/10.1016/j.fct.2022.113224.

40. Sastry, K. V. L., and P. K. Gupta. "In Vitro Inhibition of Digestive Enzymes by Heavy Metals and Their Reversal by Chelating Agent: Part I. Mercuric Chloride Intoxication." *Bulletin of Environmental Contamination and Toxicology* 20, no. 1 (July 1978): 729–735. https://doi.org/10.1007/bf01683593.

41. Carvalho, Leonardo V., Sandra S. Hacon, Claudia M. Vega, João A. Vieira, Ana L. Larentis, Rosane C. O. C, Mattos, Darielly Valente, et al. "Oxidative Stress Levels Induced by Mercury Exposure in Amazon Juvenile Populations in Brazil." *International Journal of Environmental Research and Public Health* 16, no. 15 (July 27, 2019): 2682. https://doi.org/10.3390/ijerph16152682.

42. Henriques, M. C., S. Loureiro, M. Fardilha, and M. T. Herdeiro. "Exposure to Mercury and Human Reproductive Health: A Systematic Review." *Reproductive Toxicology* 85 (April 2019): 93–103. https://doi.org/10.1016/j.reprotox.2019.02.012.

43. Brodkin, Eric, Ray Copes, Andre Mattman, James Kennedy, Robert Kling, and Annalee Yassi. "Lead and Mercury Exposures: Interpretation and Action." *Canadian Medical Association Journal* 176, no. 1 (December 13, 2006): 59–63. https://doi.org/10.1503/cmaj.060790.

44. Aduayom, I., F. Denizeau, and C. Jumarie. "Multiple Effects of Mercury on Cell Volume Regulation, Plasma Membrane Permeability, and Thiol Content in the Human Intestinal Cell Line Caco-2." *Cell Biology and Toxicology* 21, no. 3–4 (May 2005): 163–179. https://doi.org/10.1007/s10565-005-0157-7.

45. Houston, Mark C. "Role of Mercury Toxicity in Hypertension, Cardiovascular Disease, and Stroke." *The Journal of Clinical Hypertension* 13, no. 8 (July 11, 2011): 621–627. https://doi.org/10.1111/j.1751-7176.2011.00489.x.

46. Branco, Vasco, Michael Aschner, and Cristina Carvalho. "Neurotoxicity of Mercury: An Old Issue with Contemporary Significance." *Advances in Neurotoxicology* 5 (2021): 239–262. https://doi.org/10.1016/bs.ant.2021.01.001.

47. Elflein, John. "Chronic Disease Prevention in the U.S.—Statistics & Facts." *Statista*. December 18, 2023. Accessed April 18, 2024. https://www.statista.com/topics/8951/chronic-disease-prevention-in-the-us/#topicOverview.

48. American Heart Association News. "Cardiovascular Diseases Affect Nearly Half of American Adults, Statistics Show." www.heart.org. November 23, 2021. https://www.heart.org/en/news/2019/01/31/cardiovascular-diseases-affect-nearly-half-of-american-adults-statistics-show.

49. Hootman, Jennifer M., and Charles G. Helmick. "Projections of US Prevalence of Arthritis and Associated Activity Limitations." *Arthritis & Rheumatism* 54, no. 1 (December 29, 2005): 226–229. https://doi.org/10.1002/art.21562.

50. Centers for Disease Control and Prevention. "About Diabetes." *CDC*. Last reviewed June 27, 2023. Accessed April 18, 2024. https://www.cdc.gov/diabetes/about/?CDC_AAref_Val=https://www.cdc.gov/diabetes/basics/quick-facts.html.

51. Freeborn, Jessica. "Cancer Cases to Rise Steeply by 2050: What Are the Causes?" *Medical News Today*, February 8, 2024. https://www.medicalnewstoday.com/articles /an-estimated-35-million-new-cancer-cases-to-occur-in-2050-who-warns. Accessed April 18, 2024.

52. Benavidez, Gabriel A., Whitney E. Zahnd, and Peiyin Hung. "Chronic Disease Prevalence in the US: Sociodemographic and Geographic Variations by ZIP Code Tabulation Area." Centers for Disease Control and Prevention. February 29, 2024. https:// www.cdc.gov/pcd/issues/2024/23_0267.htm.

53. American Heart Association. "Heart Disease and Stroke Could Affect at Least 60% of Adults in U.S. by 2050." *American Heart Association News*. June 4, 2024. https:// www.heart.org/en/news/2024/06/04/heart-disease-and-stroke-could-affect-at-least -60-percent-of-adults-in-us-by-2050.

54. United Nations. "Chronic Diseases Taking 'Immense and Increasing Toll on Lives,' Warns WHO." *UN News*. May 19, 2023. https://news.un.org/en/story/2023/05 /1136832.

55. Partnership to Fight Chronic Disease. "The Growing Crisis of Chronic Disease in the US." Accessed August 5, 2024. https://www.fightchronicdisease.org/sites/default /files/docs/GrowingCrisisofChronicDiseaseintheUSfactsheet_81009.pdf.

56. ScienceDaily. "Population Shifts, Risk Factors May Triple U.S. Cardiovascular Disease Costs by 2050." *ScienceDaily*. June 4, 2024. https://www.sciencedaily.com /releases/2024/06/240604132105.htm.

57. Weir, Hannah K., Trevor D. Thompson, Sherri L. Stewart, and Mary C. White. "Cancer Incidence Projections in the United States Between 2015 and 2050." *Preventing Chronic Disease* 18 (2021). https://www.cdc.gov/pcd/issues/2021/21_0006 .htm.

58. Ambrose, C. "Minerals for Detoxification Support." *CASI.org*. June 13, 2023. Accessed April 18, 2024. https://www.casi.org/minerals-for-detoxification-support.

59. Melnick, J. G., K. Yurkerwich, and G. Parkin. "On the Chalcogenophilicity of Mercury: Evidence for a Strong Hg–Se Bond in [TmBut]HgSePh and Its Relevance to the Toxicity of Mercury." *Journal of the American Chemical Society* 132, no. 2 (December 18, 2009): 647–655. https://doi.org/10.1021/ja907523x.

60. Jozefczak, M., T. Remans, J. Vangronsveld, and A. Cuypers. "Glutathione Is a Key Player in Metal-Induced Oxidative Stress Defenses." *International Journal of Molecular Sciences* 13, no. 3 (March 7, 2012): 3145–3175. https://doi.org/10.3390 /ijms13033145.

61. Tang, S., X. Yu, and C. Wu. "Comparison of the Levels of Five Heavy Metals in Human Urine and Sweat after Strenuous Exercise by ICP-MS." *Journal of Applied Mathematics and Physics* 4, no. 2 (2016): 183–188. https://doi.org/10.4236/jamp .2016.42022.

62. Ibid.

63. Kuan, W. H., Y. L. Chen, and C. L. Liu. "Excretion of Ni, Pb, Cu, As, and Hg in Sweat under Two Sweating Conditions." *International Journal of Environmental*

Research and Public Health 19, no. 7 (April 4, 2022): 4323. https://doi.org/10.3390/ijerph19074323.

64. Genuis, Stephen J., Sanjay Beesoon, Daniel Birkholz, and Robert A. Lobo. "Human Excretion of Bisphenol A: Blood, Urine, and Sweat (BUS) Study." *Journal of Environmental and Public Health* 2012 (2012): 1–10. https://doi.org/10.1155/2012/185731.

65. InformedHealth.org. "Overview: Irritable Bowel Syndrome." Cologne, Germany: Institute for Quality and Efficiency in Health Care (IQWiG), 2006–. Last modified February 27, 2023. https://www.ncbi.nlm.nih.gov/books/NBK279416/.

66. Nicholson, Daniel J. "Is the Cell Really a Machine?" *Journal of Theoretical Biology* 477 (2019): 108–126. https://doi.org/10.1016/j.jtbi.2019.06.002.

67. Khoyratty, Tanweer E., Felix C. Richter, and Irina Udalova. "Macrophages: The Good, the Bad, and the Gluttony." *Frontiers in Immunology* 12 (2021): 708186. Accessed August 7, 2024. https://www.frontiersin.org/journals/immunology/articles/10.3389/fimmu.2021.708186/full.

68. Perkins, Joe. "A Holistic View of the Cell." *Latecomer Magazine*. April 24, 2023. https://latecomermag.com/article/a-holistic-view-of-the-cell/.

69. Cooper, Geoffrey M. *The Cell: A Molecular Approach*, 2nd ed. Sunderland, MA: Sinauer Associates, 2000. "Signaling in Development and Differentiation." Available from https://www.ncbi.nlm.nih.gov/books/NBK9918/.

70. Ackerman, Sandra. *Discovering the Brain*. Washington, DC: National Academies Press (US), 1992. "The Development and Shaping of the Brain." Available from https://www.ncbi.nlm.nih.gov/books/NBK234146/.

71. Kanemaki, M., H. O. Shimizu, H. Inujima, T. Miyake, and K. Shimizu. "Analysis of Red Blood Cell Movement in Whole Blood Exposed to DC and ELF Electric Fields." *Bioelectromagnetics* 43, no. 3 (April 2022): 149–159. https://doi.org/10.1002/bem.22395. PMID: 35315542; PMCID: PMC9313574.

72. Agapakis, Christina. "Is DNA Hardware or Software?" Grow by Ginkgo. June 16, 2024. https://www.growbyginkgo.com/2020/06/29/is-dna-hardware-or-software/.

73. Park, Bum Jin, Yuko Tsunetsugu, Tamami Kasetani, Takahide Kagawa, and Yoshifumi Miyazaki. "The Physiological Effects of Shinrin-yoku (Taking in the Forest Atmosphere or Forest Bathing): Evidence from Field Experiments in 24 Forests Across Japan." *Environmental Health and Preventive Medicine* 15, no. 1 (2010): 18–26. https://doi.org/10.1007/s12199-009-0086-9.

74. Li, Qing, Koichiro Morimoto, Minoru Kobayashi, Hiroshi Inagaki, Masako Katsumata, Yoshifumi Hirata, Katsuhiko Hirata, Toshifumi Shimizu, Yoshihiko J. Li, Yoshiko Wakayama, Toshio Kawada, Toyohiko Ohira, Nobuaki Takayama, and Yoshifumi Miyazaki. "A Forest Bathing Trip Increases Human Natural Killer Activity and Expression of Anti-cancer Proteins in Female Subjects." *Journal of Biological Regulators and Homeostatic Agents* 22, no. 1 (2008): 45–55. https://pubmed.ncbi.nlm.nih.gov/18394317/.

75. Lambert, Guillaume W., Michael J. Reid, Geoffrey F. Kaye, Eugene K. Jennings, and Felix A. Esler. "Effect of Sunlight and Season on Serotonin Turnover in the Brain." *The Lancet* 360, no. 9348 (2002): 1840–1842. https://doi.org/10.1016/S0140-6736(02)11737-5.

76. Smithsonian Tropical Research Institute. "Connections in Nature: Plants, Animals, Microbes, and Environments." Accessed May 19, 2024. https://stri.si.edu/research -theme/connections-nature-plants-animals-microbes-and-environments.

77. Ibid.

78. McCrory, C., M. Meaney, and K. J. O'Donnell. "The Legacy of Early Life Stress on the Epigenome: Mechanisms, Phenotypic Consequences, and Possibilities for Intervention." *National Center for Biotechnology Information.* Published December 2021. Accessed August 7, 2024. https://www.ncbi.nlm.nih.gov/pmc/articles /PMC8848501/.

79. Niccoli, Teresa, and Linda Partridge. "Ageing as a Risk Factor for Disease." *Current Biology* 22, no. 17 (September 11, 2012): R741–52. https://doi.org/10.1016/j.cub .2012.07.024. PMID: 22975005.

80. National Human Genome Research Institute. "Epigenome." *Genetics Home Reference.* Accessed May 19, 2024. https://www.genome.gov/genetics-glossary/Epigenome.

81. Davis, Josh. "Scientists Grow Flatworm with Two Heads Instead of Tail." *IFLScience.* Accessed May 19, 2024. https://www.iflscience.com/scientists-grow-flatworm-with -two-heads-instead-of-tail-41823.

82. Harvard Medical School. "Loss of Epigenetic Information Can Drive Aging, Restoration Can Reverse It." Accessed May 19, 2024. https://hms.harvard.edu/news/loss -epigenetic-information-can-drive-aging-restoration-can-reverse.

83. Sherman, Bennett M. "David Sinclair: DNA Tagging, Rather Than DNA Damage, Drives Aging and Is Reversible." NAD.com. January 2, 2024. https://www.nad.com /news/harvard-professor-david-sinclairs-information-theory-of-aging.

84. Mullard, Asher. "The Yamanaka Recipe for Making Young Cells." *Nature Biotechnology* 40 (2022): 125–128. https://doi.org/10.1038/d41587-022-00002-4.

85. Impact Journals. "Discovery of Chemical Means to Reverse Aging and Restore Cellular Function." Phys.org. July 13, 2023. https://phys.org/news/2023-07-discovery -chemical-reverse-aging-cellular.html.

86. Ibid.

87. Grow by Ginkgo. "Is DNA Hardware or Software?" *Grow by Ginkgo.* June 29, 2020. https://www.growbyginkgo.com/2020/06/29/is-dna-hardware-or-software/.

88. Peixoto, Paul, Pierre-François Cartron, Aurélien A. Serandour, and Eric Hervouet. "From 1957 to Nowadays: A Brief History of Epigenetics." *International Journal of Molecular Sciences* 21, no. 20 (2020): 7571. https://doi.org/10.3390/ijms 21207571.

89. Haker, Helene, Wolfgang Kawohl, Uwe Herwig, and Wulf Rössler. "Mirror Neuron Activity During Contagious Yawning—An fMRI Study." *Brain Imaging and Behavior* 7, no. 1 (March 2013): 28–34. https://doi.org/10.1007/s11682-012-9189-9. PMID: 22772979.

90. National Human Genome Research Institute. "Epigenomics Fact Sheet." *National Human Genome Research Institute.* Last modified October 5, 2023. https://www .genome.gov/about-genomics/fact-sheets/Epigenomics-Fact-Sheet.

91. Harvard Medical School. "What Is Epigenetics?" *Harvard Medical School News,* December 5, 2019. https://hms.harvard.edu/news/what-epigenetics.

92. Sinclair, David A. and Lenny Guarente. "Aging: Why Do We Age?" *Nature Reviews Genetics* 15 (2014): 563–578. https://doi.org/10.1038/nrg3771.

93. Pal, Sunil, and Mirza S. Baig. "DNA Methylation: An Epigenetic Mechanism with the Potential for Therapeutic Interventions." *Progress in Molecular Biology and Translational Science* 173 (2020): 151–185. https://doi.org/10.1016/bs.pmbts.2020.01.003.

94. Ibid.

95. Melore, Chris. "Survey: 53% of Americans Admit They're Not Living a 'Healthy' Lifestyle." Study Finds. April 7, 2022. https://studyfinds.org/healthy-lifestyle-income/.

96. Jain, Vartika. "What Is Modern Medicine." IGI Global. 2020. https://www.igi-global.com/dictionary/a-review-of-traditional-medicinal-plants-used-for-treatment-of-leucorrhoea-in-india/85153.

97. IGI Global. "A Review of Traditional Medicinal Plants Used for Treatment of Leucorrhoea in India." Accessed May 19, 2024. https://www.igi-global.com/dictionary/a-review-of-traditional-medicinal-plants-used-for-treatment-of-leucorrhoea-in-india/85153.

98. Tulchinsky, Theodore H. and Elena A. Varavikova. "A History of Public Health." *The New Public Health* 10 (October 2014): 1–42. https://www.ncbi.nlm.nih.gov/pmc/articles/PMC7170188/.

99. World Health Organization. "Traditional Medicine Has a Long History of Contributing to Conventional Medicine and Continues to Hold Promise." Accessed May 19, 2024. https://www.who.int/news-room/feature-stories/detail/traditional-medicine-has-a-long-history-of-contributing-to-conventional-medicine-and-continues-to-hold-promise.

100. Ventola, C. Lee. "Current Issues Regarding Complementary and Alternative Medicine (CAM) in the United States: Part 1: The Widespread Use of CAM and the Need for Better-Informed Health Care Professionals to Provide Patient Counseling." *Pharmacy and Therapeutics* 35, no. 8 (August 2010): 461–468. PMID: 20844696; PMCID: PMC2935644.

101. Vedam, Raj, Tarun A. Pansare, and Jagat Narula. "Contributions of Ancient Indian Knowledge to Modern Medicine and Cardiology." *Indian Heart Journal* 73, no. 5 (September–October 2021): 531–534.. Epub September 16, 2021. PMID: 34627563; PMCID: PMC8514395. https://doi.org/10.1016/j.ihj.2021.09.010

102. Lu, Weidong, Elizabeth Dean-Clower, Anne Doherty-Gilman, and David S. Rosenthal. "The Value of Acupuncture in Cancer Care." *Hematology/oncology clinics of North America* 22, no. 4 (August 2008): 631–viii. https://www.ncbi.nlm.nih.gov/pmc/articles/PMC2642987/.

103. Hewlings, Susan J., and Douglas S. Kalman. "Curcumin: A Review of Its Effects on Human Health." *Foods* 6, no. 10 (October 2022): 92. https://pubmed.ncbi.nlm.nih.gov/29065496/.

104. Ibid.

105. Dubey, Roshan Kumar, Satyam Shukla, Zeashan Hussain, and Mohammad Tasin. "A Systematic Review of the Pharmacological and Phytochemical Profiles of Madagascar Periwinkle as Potential Dietary Supplement." *Chinese Journal of Applied Physiology* (2023): 39:e20230002. https://pubmed.ncbi.nlm.nih.gov/38651238/.

106. Kairey, Lana, Tamara Agnew, Esther Joy Bowles, Bronwyn J. Barkla, Jon Wardle, and Romy Lauche. "Efficacy and Safety of Melaleuca Alternifolia (Tea Tree) Oil for Human Health-A Systematic Review of Randomized Controlled Trials." *Frontiers in Pharmacology* 14 (2023). https://doi.org/10.3389/fphar.2023.1116077.

107. Yan, Li-Shan, Brian Chi-Yan Cheng, Shuo-Feng Zhang, Gan Luo, Chao Zhang, Qing-Gao Wang, Xiu-Qiong Fu, Yi-Wei Wang, and Yi Zhang. "Tibetan Medicine for Diabetes Mellitus: Overview of Pharmacological Perspectives." *Frontiers in Pharmacology* 12 (2021). https://www.ncbi.nlm.nih.gov/pmc/articles/PMC 8566911/.

108. Yim, Tae-Bin, Gyu-Ri Jeon, Hye-Jin Lee, Kyeong-Hwa Lee, Hye-Min Heo, Han-Gyul Lee, Seungwon Kwon, et al. "The Effectiveness of Kami Guibi-Tang for Cognitive Impairment Patients: A Retrospective Chart Review." *Heliyon* 10, no. 1 (2023): e23615. https://pubmed.ncbi.nlm.nih.gov/38187321/.

109. Merali, Zul, Christian Cayer, Pamela Kent, Rui Liu, Cory S. Harris, and John T. Arnason. "Sacred Maya Incense, Copal (Protium Copal—Burseraceae), Has Anti-anxiety Effects in Animal Models." *Journal of Ethnopharmacology* 216 (2018): 63–70. https://pubmed.ncbi.nlm.nih.gov/29414121/.

110. Guasch-Ferre, M., and W. C. Willett. "The Mediterranean Diet and Health: A Comprehensive Overview." *Journal of Internal Medicine* 290, no. 3 (2021): 549–566. https://pubmed.ncbi.nlm.nih.gov/34423871/.

111. "Exhausted Nation: Americans More Tired than Ever, Survey Finds." Safety+Health RSS. February 3, 2022. https://www.safetyandhealthmagazine.com/articles/22112 -exhausted-nation-americans-more-tired-than-ever-survey-finds.

112. "How Does Caffeine Give US Energy?" Friedman School of Nutrition Science and Policy. September 8, 2022. https://nutrition.tufts.edu/news/how-does-caffeine-give -us-energy.

113. Brand, M. D., A. L. Orr, I. V. Perevoshchikova, and C. L. Quinlan. "The Role of Mitochondrial Function and Cellular Bioenergetics in Ageing and Disease." *The British Journal of Dermatology* 169, no. 2 (2013): 1–8. https://www.ncbi.nlm.nih.gov /pmc/articles/PMC4321783/.

114. "Mitochondrion—Much More than an Energy Converter." British Society for Cell Biology. Accessed May 20, 2024. https://bscb.org/learning-resources/softcell -e-learning/mitochondrion-much-more-than-an-energy-converter/.

115. Wakim, Suzanne and Mandeep Grewal. "5.9: Cellular Respiration." Biology LibreTexts. September 4, 2021. https://bio.libretexts.org/Bookshelves/Human _Biology/Human_Biology_(Wakim_and_Grewal)/05%3A_Cells/5.09%3A_Cellular _Respiration.

116. Eberle, Suzanne Girard. "The Body's Fuel Sources." Human Kinetics. Accessed May 20, 2024. https://us.humankinetics.com/blogs/excerpt/the-bodys-fuel-sources.

117. "Autoimmune Diseases." National Institute of Environmental Health Sciences. Accessed May 20, 2024. https://www.niehs.nih.gov/health/topics/conditions /autoimmune.

118. Gore, A. C., V. A. Chappell, S. E. Fenton, J. A. Flaws, A. Nadal, G. S. Prins, J. Toppari, and R. T. Zoeller. "EDC-2: The Endocrine Society's Second Scientific

Statement on Endocrine-Disrupting Chemicals." *Endocrine Reviews* 36, no. 6 (2015): E1–E150. https://pubmed.ncbi.nlm.nih.gov/26544531/.; Safaris, Stravos, Vasilis P. Androutsopoulos, Aristeidis M. Tsatsakis, and Demetrios A. Spandidos. "Human Exposure to Endocrine Disrupting Chemicals: Effects on the Male and Female Reproductive Systems." *Environmental Toxicology and Pharmacology* 51 (2017): 56–70. https://pubmed.ncbi.nlm.nih.gov/28292651/.

119. Cao, Xinxi, Yangyang Cheng, Chenjie Xu Xu, Yabing Hou, Hongxi Yang, Shu Li, Ying Gao, Peng Jia, and Yaogang Wang. "Risk of Accidents or Chronic Disorders from Improper Use of Mobile Phones: A Systematic Review and Meta-Analysis." *Journal of Medical Internet Research* 24, no 1 (2022): e21313. https://pubmed.ncbi.nlm.nih.gov/35049511/; Ye, Ziliang, Yanjun Zhang, Yuanyuan Zhang, Sisi Yang, Mengzi Liu, Qimeng Wu, Chun Zhou, Panpan He, Xiaoqin Gan, and Xianhui Qin. "Mobile Phone Calls, Genetic Susceptibility, and New-Onset Hypertension: Results from 212 046 UK Biobank Participants." *European Heart Journal—Digital Health* 4, no. 3 (2023): 165–174. https://pubmed.ncbi.nlm.nih.gov/37265874/.

120. Mitchell, Diane C., Carol A. Knight, Jon Hockenberry, Robyn Teplansky, and Terryl J. Hartman. "Beverage Caffeine Intakes in the U.S." *Food and Chemical Toxicology* 63 (2014): 136–142. https://pubmed.ncbi.nlm.nih.gov/24189158/.

121. Bosiacki, M., M. Tarnowski, K. Misiakiewicz-Has, and A. Lubkowska. "The Effect of Cold-Water Swimming on Energy Metabolism, Dynamics, and Mitochondrial Biogenesis in the Muscles of Aging Rats." *International Journal of Molecular Sciences* 25, no. 7 (April 5, 2024): 4055. https://doi.org/10.3390/ijms25074055.

122. Hayes, Tara O'Neill and Katerina Kerska. "Primer: Agriculture Subsidies and Their Influence on the Composition of U.S. Food Supply and Consumption." AAF. November 3, 2021. https://www.americanactionforum.org/research/primer-agriculture-subsidies-and-their-influence-on-the-composition-of-u-s-food-supply-and-consumption/; Schultz, James. "Albert Szent-Gyorgyi Vitamin C—Landmark." American Chemical Society. 2002. https://www.acs.org/education/whatischemistry/landmarks/szentgyorgyi.html.

123. Hopkins, F. Gowland. *The Earlier History of the Vitamin.* HathiTrust Digital Library. Accessed November 3, 2024. https://babel.hathitrust.org/cgi/pt?id=mdp.39015069802166&view=1up&seq=353&q1=vitamine.

124. Backstrand, J. R.. "The History and Future of Food Fortification in the United States: A Public Health Perspective." *Nutrition Reviews* 60, no. 1 (2002): 15–26. https://pubmed.ncbi.nlm.nih.gov/11842999/.

125. Mozaffarian, Dariush, Irwin Rosenberg, and Ricardo Uauy. "History of Modern Nutrition Science—Implications for Current Research, Dietary Guidelines, and Food Policy." *BMJ* 361 (2018): k2392. https://www.ncbi.nlm.nih.gov/pmc/articles/PMC5998735/.

126. Kearns, Cristin E., Laura A. Schmidt, and Stanton A. Glantz. "Sugar Industry and Coronary Heart Disease Research: A Historical Analysis of Internal Industry Documents." *JAMA Internal Medicine* 176, no. 11 (2016): 1680–1685. https://pubmed.ncbi.nlm.nih.gov/27617709/.

127. Carpenter, Kenneth J. *Protein and Energy: A Study of Changing Ideas in Nutrition.* Accessed May 21, 2024. https://books.google.com/books?hl=en&lr=&id=GtQT hfnhKLsC&oi.

128. Mozaffarian, Dariush, Irwin Rosenberg, and Ricardo Uauy. "History of Modern Nutrition Science—Implications for Current Research, Dietary Guidelines, and Food Policy." *BMJ* 361 (2018): k2392. https://www.ncbi.nlm.nih.gov/pmc/articles /PMC5998735/.

129. Mente, Andrew, Lawrence de Koning, Harry S. Shannon, and Sonia S. Anand. "A Systematic Review of the Evidence Supporting a Causal Link Between Dietary Factors and Coronary Heart Disease." *Archives of Internal Medicine* 169, no. 7 (2009): 659–669. https://pubmed.ncbi.nlm.nih.gov/19364995/.

130. Mozaffarian, Dariush. "Dietary and Policy Priorities for Cardiovascular Disease, Diabetes, and Obesity: A Comprehensive Review." *Circulation* 133, no. 2 (2016): 187–225. https://pubmed.ncbi.nlm.nih.gov/26746178/.

131. "Visualizing Dietary Guidelines: A Brief History of the Food Pyramid." Knight Lab. Accessed August 15, 2024. https://cdn.knightlab.com/libs/timeline3/latest /embed/index.html?source=1APsK4V8nJVeowWSAOTu-NgCVOZifQYCd -FH3Ks1DdKM.

132. Wikipedia, s.v. "Food Pyramid (Nutrition)." Last modified August 18, 2023. https:// en.wikipedia.org/wiki/Food_pyramid_(nutrition).

133. Hayes, Tara O'Neill and Katerina Kerska. "Primer: Agriculture Subsidies and Their Influence on the Composition of U.S. Food Supply and Consumption." AAF. November 3, 2021. https://www.americanactionforum.org/research/primer -agriculture-subsidies-and-their-influence-on-the-composition-of-u-s-food-supply -and-consumption/; Schultz, James. "Albert Szent-Gyorgyi Vitamin C—Landmark." American Chemical Society. 2002.

134. Dodds, W. J. "Central Nervous System Regulation of Appetite in Humans and Pet Animals." *Annals of Clinical and xperimental Metabolism* 2, no. 1 (1970): 1013. https://doi.org/10.47739/2572-2492/1013.

135. Ahima, Rexford S., and Daniel A. Antwi. "Brain Regulation of Appetite and Satiety." *Endocrinology and Metabolism Clinics of North America* 37, no. 4 (2008): 811–823. https://www.ncbi.nlm.nih.gov/pmc/articles/PMC2710609/.

136. Dodds, W. J. "Central Nervous System Regulation of Appetite in Humans and Pet Animals." *Annals of Clinical and xperimental Metabolism* 2, no. 1 (1970): 1013. https://doi.org/10.47739/2572-2492/1013.

137. Campbell, T. Colin. *Whole: Rethinking the Science of Nutrition.* BenBella Books, 2013; Fuhrman, Joel. "The Hidden Dangers of Fast and Processed Food." *American Journal of Lifestyle Medicine* 12, no. 5 (2018): 375–381. https://www.ncbi.nlm.nih .gov/pmc/articles/PMC6146358/; Fuhrman, Joel. "Beginner's Guide to the Nutritarian Diet." Dr. Fuhrman (blog). Accessed May 21, 2024. https://www.drfuhrman .com/blog/210/beginners-guide.

138. Monteiro, Carlos A., Geoffrey Cannon, Renata B. Levy, Jean-Claude Moubarac, Maria Lc Louzada, Fernanda Rauber, Neha Khandpur, et al. "Ultra-Processed

Foods: What They Are and How to Identify Them." *Public Health Nutrition* 22, no. 5 (2019): 936–941. https://pubmed.ncbi.nlm.nih.gov/30744710/.

139. "Fooddata Central Search Results." FoodData Central. Accessed May 21, 2024. https://fdc.nal.usda.gov/fdc-app.html#/food-search?query=&type=Foundation.

140. "Vitamin C (Ascorbic Acid)." Mount Sinai Health System. Accessed May 21, 2024. https://www.mountsinai.org/health-library/supplement/vitamin-c-ascorbic-acid.

141. "Selenium." The Nutrition Source. May 9, 2024. https://nutritionsource.hsph.harvard .edu/selenium/.

142. Spreadbury, Ian. "Comparison with Ancestral Diets Suggests Dense Acellular Carbohydrates Promote an Inflammatory Microbiota, and May Be the Primary Dietary Cause of Leptin Resistance and Obesity." *Diabetes, Metabolic Syndrome and Obesity: Targets and Therapy* 5 (2012): 175–198. https://www.ncbi.nlm.nih.gov/pmc/articles /PMC3402009/.

143. "Rethinking Fructose in Your Diet." Harvard Health. July 1, 2013. https://www .health.harvard.edu/staying-healthy/rethinking-fructose-in-your-diet.

144. Fuhrman, Joel. "The Hidden Dangers of Fast and Processed Food." *American Journal of Lifestyle Medicine* 12, no. 5 (2018): 375–381. https://www.ncbi.nlm.nih.gov/pmc /articles/PMC6146358/; Fuhrman, Joel. "Beginner's Guide to the Nutritarian Diet." Dr. Fuhrman (blog). Accessed May 21, 2024. https://www.drfuhrman.com/blog/210 /beginners-guide.

145. Espinosa-Salas, S. and M. Gonzalez-Arias. "Nutrition: Micronutrient Intake, Imbalances, and Interventions." Last updated September 21, 2023. In *StatPearls [Internet]*. Treasure Island, FL: StatPearls Publishing. January 2024. https://www.ncbi.nlm.nih .gov/books/NBK597352/.

146. Stryer, Lubert, Jeremy M. Berg, John L. Tymoczko, and Gregory J. Gatto Jr. *Biochemistry*. 5th ed. New York: W.H. Freeman, 2002. https://www.ncbi.nlm.nih.gov /books/NBK9879/.

147. Alberts, Bruce, Alexander Johnson, Julian Lewis, et al. *Molecular Biology of the Cell*. 4th ed. New York: Garland Science, 2002. https://www.ncbi.nlm.nih.gov/books /NBK9921/.

148. Puertollano, M. A., E. Puertollano, G. Á. de Cienfuegos, and M. A. de Pablo. "Dietary Antioxidants: Immunity and Host Defense." *Current Topics in Medicinal Chemistry* 11, no. 14 (2011): 1752–66. https://doi.org/10.2174/156802611796235107.

149. Mitra, S., S. Paul, S. Roy, H. Sutradhar, T. Bin Emran, F. Nainu, M. U. Khandaker, M. Almalki, P. Wilairatana, and M. S. Mubarak. "Exploring the Immune-Boosting Functions of Vitamins and Minerals as Nutritional Food Bioactive Compounds: A Comprehensive Review." *Molecules* 27, no. 2 (2022): 555. https://doi.org/10.3390 /molecules27020555.

150. Santana-Gálvez, J., J. Villela-Castrejón, S. O. Serna-Saldívar, L. Cisneros-Zevallos, and D. A. Jacobo-Velázquez. "Synergistic Combinations of Curcumin, Sulforaphane, and Dihydrocaffeic Acid Against Human Colon Cancer Cells." *International Journal of Molecular Sciences* 21, no. 9 (April 28, 2020): 3108. https://doi.org/10.3390 /ijms21093108.

151. Daryanavard, H., A. E. Postiglione, J. K. Mühlemann, and G. K. Muday. "Flavonols Modulate Plant Development, Signaling, and Stress Responses." *Current Opinion in Plant Biology* 72 (April 2023): 102350. https://doi.org/10.1016/j.pbi.2023.102350.

152. Harmon, Brook E., Melinda Forthofer, Erin O. Bantum, and Claudio R. Nigg. "Perceived Influence and College Students' Diet and Physical Activity Behaviors: An Examination of Ego-Centric Social Networks." *BMC Public Health* 16 (2016): 473. https://www.ncbi.nlm.nih.gov/pmc/articles/PMC4895992/; Lynn, Theo, Pierangelo Rosati, Guto Leoni Santos, and Patricia Takako Endo. "Sorting the Healthy Diet Signal from the Social Media Expert Noise: Preliminary Evidence from the Healthy Diet Discourse on Twitter." *International Journal of Environmental Research and Public Health* 17, no. 22 (2020): 8557. https://www.ncbi.nlm.nih.gov/pmc/articles /PMC7698912/.

153. Erenstein, O., M. Jaleta, K. A. Mottaleb, K. Sonder, J. Donovan, and H. J. Braun. "Global Trends in Wheat Production, Consumption and Trade." In *Wheat Improvement*, edited by M. P. Reynolds and H. J. Braun. Cham: Springer, 2022. https://doi .org/10.1007/978-3-030-90673-3_4.

154. International Grains Council. "Home." *International Grains Council.* Accessed August 13, 2024. https://www.igc.int/en/default.aspx.

155. Jain, Vartika. "What Is Modern Medicine." IGI Global. 2020. https://www.igi -global.com/dictionary/a-review-of-traditional-medicinal-plants-used-for-treatment -of-leucorrhoea-in-india/85153.

156. Holesh, Julie E., Sanah Aslam, and Andrew Martin. *Physiology, Carbohydrates*. In *StatPearls [Internet]*. Treasure Island, FL: StatPearls Publishing. January 2024 https:// pubmed.ncbi.nlm.nih.gov/29083823/.

157. Okamura, Tomonori, Kazuhisa Tsukamoto, Hidenori Arai, Yoshio Fujioka, Yasushi Ishigaki, et al. "Japan Atherosclerosis Society (JAS) Guidelines for Prevention of Atherosclerotic Cardiovascular Diseases 2022." *Journal of Atherosclerosis and Thrombosis* 31, no. 6 (2024): 641–853. https://doi.org/10.5551/jat.GL2022.

158. Hu, Y., W. C. Willett, J. A. E. Manson, B. Rosner, F. B. Hu, and Q. Sun. "Intake of Whole Grain Foods and Risk of Coronary Heart Disease in US Men and Women." *BMC Medicine* 20, no. 1 (June 10, 2022): 192. https://doi.org/10.1186/s12916-022 -02396-z.

159. Della Pepa, G., C. Vetrani, M. Vitale, and G. Riccardi. "Wholegrain Intake and Risk of Type 2 Diabetes: Evidence from Epidemiological and Intervention Studies." *Nutrients* 10, no. 9 (September 12, 2018): 1288. https://doi.org/10.3390/nu10091288.

160. Aune, D., N. Keum, E. Giovannucci, L. T. Fadnes, P. Boffetta, D. C. Greenwood, et al. "Whole Grain Consumption and Risk of Cardiovascular Disease, Cancer, and All-Cause and Cause-Specific Mortality: Systematic Review and Dose-Response Meta-Analysis of Prospective Studies." *BMJ* 353 (2016): i2716. https://doi.org/10 .1136/bmj.i2716.

161. Um, C. Y., B. A. Peters, H. S. Choi, P. Oberstein, D. B. Beggs, M. Usyk, F. Wu, R. B. Hayes, S. M. Gapstur, M. L. McCullough, and J. Ahn. "Grain, Gluten, and Dietary Fiber Intake Influence Gut Microbial Diversity: Data from the Food and

Microbiome Longitudinal Investigation." *Cancer Research Communications* 3, no. 1 (January 11, 2023): 43–53. https://doi.org/10.1158/2767-9764.CRC-22-0154.

162. Biesiekierski, Jessica R. "What is Gluten?" *Journal of Gastroenterology and Hepatology* 32, no. S1 (2017): 78–81. https://doi.org/10.1111/jgh.13703.

163. Almarshad, Mohammed I., Rayan Algonaiman, Hala F. Alharbi, Maha S. Almujay-dil, and Hazem Barakat. "Relationship Between Ultra-Processed Food Consumption and Risk of Diabetes Mellitus: A Mini-Review." *Nutrients* 14, no. 12 (2022): 2366. https://doi.org/10.3390/nu14122366.

164. Monteiro, Carlos Augusto, Geoffrey Cannon, Renata Bertazzi Levy, Maria Laura da Costa Louzada, and Jean-Claude Moubarac. "Ultra-Processed Foods: What They Are and How to Identify Them." *Public Health Nutrition* 22, no. 5 (2019): 936–941. https://doi.org/10.1017/S1368980018003762.

165. International Agency for Research on Cancer (IARC), World Health Organization. *IARC Monographs Volume 112: Evaluation of Five Organophosphate Insecticides and Herbicides*. 2015.

166. Mesnage, Robin, and Michael N. Antoniou. "Facts and Fallacies in the Debate on Glyphosate Toxicity." *Frontiers in Public Health* 5 (2017): 316. https://doi.org/10.3389/fpubh.2017.00316.

167. Gobbetti, Marco, Maria De Angelis, Paola Di Cagno, Mauro Minervini, Maria Teresa Rizzello. "Sourdough Bread Making with Lactobacilli: A Tool for the Improved Nutritional Quality of Wheat Flours." *Journal of Cereal Science* 56, no. 2 (2012): 232–240. https://doi.org/10.1016/j.jcs.2012.02.007.

168. Baranski, Marcin, Dominika Średnicka-Tober, Nicola Scialabba, Chris Seal, Roy Sanderson, Charles Benbrook, Gavin Stewart, et al. "Higher Antioxidant and Lower Cadmium Concentrations and Lower Incidence of Pesticide Residues in Organically Grown Crops: A Systematic Literature Review and Meta-Analyses." *British Journal of Nutrition* 112, no. 5 (2014): 794–811. https://doi.org/10.1017/S0007114514001366.

169. Monteiro, Carlos A., Geoffrey Cannon, Renata B. Levy, Maria L. C. Louzada, Jean-Claude Moubarac. "Ultra-Processed Foods: What They Are and How to Identify Them." *Public Health Nutrition* 22, no. 5 (2019): 936–941. https://doi.org/10.1017/S1368980018003762.

170. Polak, Rani, Edward M. Phillips, and Amy Campbell. "Legumes: Health Benefits and Culinary Approaches to Increase Intake." *Clinical Diabetes: A Publication of the American Diabetes Association* 33, no. 4 (2015): 198–205. https://www.ncbi.nlm.nih.gov/pmc/articles/PMC4608274/.

171. Mudryj, Adriana N., Nancy L. Yu, and Alexandra M. Aukema. "Nutritional and Health Benefits of Pulses." *Applied Physiology, Nutrition, and Metabolism* 39, no. 11 (2014): 1197–1204. https://doi.org/10.1139/apnm-2013-0557.

172. Rebello, C. J., R.A. Beyl, J.P. Lomenick, K. Kloiber, W. Xie, W.D. Johnson, and F.L. Greenway. "Effect of a Phase 2 Starch Neutralizer on Body Weight after Eight Weeks of Multiple Doses in Healthy Overweight Adults: A Randomized, Double-Blind, Placebo-Controlled Study." *Nutrients* 7, no. 7 (2015): 4774–4786. https://doi.org/10.3390/nu7074774.

173. Anderson, James W., Patricia Baird, Rhonda H. Davis, Shaomei Ferreri, Mary Knudtson, Alison Koraym, Valerie Waters, and Cheryl L. Williams. "Health Benefits of Dietary Fiber." *Nutrition Reviews* 67, no. 4 (2009): 188–205. https://doi.org/10 .1111/j.1753-4887.2009.00189.x.

174. Messina, Valerie. "Nutritional and Health Benefits of Dried Beans." *The American Journal of Clinical Nutrition* 76, no. 3 (2002): 437–442. https://doi.org/10.1093/ajcn /76.3.437.

175. Ranilla, L. G M.I. Genovese, and F.M. Lajolo. "Polyphenols and Antioxidant Capacity of Seed Coat and Cotyledon from a Brazilian Cultivar of Common Bean (Phaseolus vulgaris L.) Before and After Cooking." *Journal of Agricultural and Food Chemistry* 55, no. 15 (2007): 3940–3949. https://doi.org/10.1021/jf0 73113k.

176. Siddhuraju, P. and K. Becker. "Effect of Various Domestic Processing Methods on Antinutrients and in Vitro Protein and Starch Digestibility of Two Indigenous Varieties of Indian Tribal Pulse, Mucuna pruriens var. utilis." *Journal of the Science of Food and Agriculture* 80, no. 14 (2000): 2061–2070. https://doi.org/10.1002/1097 -0010(200011)80:14<2061::AID-JSFA736>3.0.CO;2-L.

177. Nkhata, S. G., E. Ayua, E. H. Kamau, and J. B. Shingiro. "Fermentation and Germination Improve Nutritional Value of Cereals and Legumes Through Activation of Endogenous Enzymes." *Food Science & Nutrition* 6, no. 8 (October 16, 2018): 2446–2458. https://doi.org/10.1002/fsn3.846.

178. Lynch, Sean R. and Jack S. Cook. "Interaction of Vitamin C and Iron." *Annals of the New York Academy of Sciences* 355, no. 1 (1980): 32–44. https://doi.org/10.1111/j.1749 -6632.1980.tb21325.x.

179. Slavin, Joanne L. and Beate Lloyd. "Health Benefits of Fruits and Vegetables." *Advances in Nutrition* 3, no. 4 (2012): 506–516. https://doi.org/10.3945/an.112 .002154.

180. Hyson, D. A. "A Comprehensive Review of Apples and Apple Components and Their Relationship to Human Health." *Advances in Nutrition* 2, no. 5 (2011): 408–420. https://doi.org/10.3945/an.111.000513.

181. Popkin, Barry M., Kristen E. D'Anci, and Irwin H. Rosenberg. "Water, Hydration and Health." *Nutrition Reviews* 68, no. 8 (2010): 439–458. https://doi.org/10.1111 /j.1753-4887.2010.00304.x.

182. Ludwig, David S. "The Glycemic Index: Physiological Mechanisms Relating to Obesity, Diabetes, and Cardiovascular Disease." *The Journal of the American Medical Association* 287, no. 18 (2002): 2414–2423. https://doi.org/10.1001/jama.287.18.2414.

183. McCrory, Megan A., Phyllis A. McCrory, Stephen L. Takeda, and Katherine A. Campbell. "Eating Frequency and Energy Regulation: A Physiological View." *The Journal of Nutrition* 141, no. 1 (2011): 154–157. https://doi.org/10.3945/jn.109 .114793.

184. Viroli, G., A. Kalmpourtzidou, and H. Cena. "Exploring Benefits and Barriers of Plant-Based Diets: Health, Environmental Impact, Food Accessibility and Acceptability." *Nutrients* 15, no. 22 (2023): 4723. https://doi.org/10.3390/nu15224723.

185. Ruprich, Jiri, Marie Dofkova, and Jaroslava Rehurkova. "Safety and Benefits of Lectins and Their Role in Human Nutrition." *Critical Reviews in Food Science and Nutrition* 51, no. 1 (2011): 77–85. https://doi.org/10.1080/10408390903567497.

186. Adamcová, A., K. H. Laursen, and N. Z. Ballin. "Lectin Activity in Commonly Consumed Plant-Based Foods: Calling for Method Harmonization and Risk Assessment." *Foods* 10, no. 11 (2021): 2796. https://doi.org/10.3390/foods10112796.

187. Miglio, Claudia, Enrico Chiavaro, Andrea Visconti, Valentina Fogliano, and Nicola Pellegrini. "Effects of Different Cooking Methods on Nutritional and Physicochemical Characteristics of Selected Vegetables." *Journal of Agricultural and Food Chemistry* 56, no. 1 (2008): 139–147. https://doi.org/10.1021/jf072304b.

188. Zhang, Youyou, et al. "Dietary Vegetables and Cardiometabolic Disease Risk." *Current Atherosclerosis Reports* 20, no. 11 (2018): 64. https://doi.org/10.1007/s11883-018 -0771-6.

189. "About Clint Ober." Earthing. Accessed May 21, 2024. https://www.earthing.com /pages/about-clint-ober.

190. Chevalier, Gaétan, Stephen T. Sinatra, James L. Oschman, Karol Sokal, and Pawel Sokal. "Earthing: Health Implications of Reconnecting the Human Body to the Earth's Surface Electrons." *Journal of Environmental and Public Health*, 2012. https:// www.ncbi.nlm.nih.gov/pmc/articles/PMC3265077/; Oschman, James L., Gaétan Chevalier, and Richard Brown. "The Effects of Grounding (Earthing) on Inflammation, the Immune Response, Wound Healing, and Prevention and Treatment of Chronic Inflammatory and Autoimmune Diseases." *Journal of Inflammation Research* 8 (2015): 83–96. https://www.ncbi.nlm.nih.gov/pmc/articles/PMC4378297/.

191. Forbes, Jack D. "Indigenous Americans: Spirituality and Ecos." *American Academy of Arts & Sciences* 130, no. 4 (Fall 2001): 283–300. https://www.amacad.org /publication/indigenous-americans-spirituality-and-ecos.

192. Williams, E. R. and S. J. Heckman. "The Local Diurnal Variation of Cloud Electrification and the Global Diurnal Variation of Negative Charge on the Earth." *Journal of Geophysical Research: Atmospheres* 98, no. D3 (1993): 5221–5234. https://agupubs .onlinelibrary.wiley.com/doi/abs/10.1029/92JD02642.

193. Phaniendra, Alugoju, Dinesh Babu Jestadi, and Latha Periyasamy. "Free Radicals: Properties, Sources, Targets, and Their Implication in Various Diseases." *Indian Journal of Clinical Biochemistry* 30, no. 1 (2014): 11–26. https://www.ncbi.nlm.nih.gov /pmc/articles/PMC4310837/.

194. Oschman, James L., Gaétan Chevalier, and Richard Brown. "The Effects of Grounding (Earthing) on Inflammation, the Immune Response, Wound Healing, and Prevention and Treatment of Chronic Inflammatory and Autoimmune Diseases." *Journal of Inflammation Research* 8 (2015): 83–96. https://www.ncbi.nlm.nih.gov /pmc/articles/PMC4378297/.

195. Neha, Kumari, Rafi Haider, Ankita Pathak, and M. Shahar Yar. "Medicinal Prospects of Antioxidants: A Review." *European Journal of Medicinal Chemistry* 178 (2019): 687–704. https://pubmed.ncbi.nlm.nih.gov/31228811/.

196. Furman, David, Judith Campisi, Eric Verdin, Pedro Carrera-Bastos, Sasha Targ, Claudio Franceschi, Luigi Ferrucci, et al. "Chronic Inflammation in the Etiology of

Disease across the Life Span." *Nature Medicine* 25, no. 12 (2019): 1822–1832. https://www.ncbi.nlm.nih.gov/pmc/articles/PMC7147972/.

197. Sinatra, Stephen T., Drew S. Sinatra, Stephen W. Sinatra, and Gaetan Chevalier. "Grounding—the Universal Anti-Inflammatory Remedy." *Biomedical Journal* 46, no. 1 (2023): 11–16. https://www.ncbi.nlm.nih.gov/pmc/articles/PMC10105021/.

198. Oschman, James L., Gaétan Chevalier, and Richard Brown. "The Effects of Grounding (Earthing) on Inflammation, the Immune Response, Wound Healing, and Prevention and Treatment of Chronic Inflammatory and Autoimmune Diseases." *Journal of Inflammation Research* 8 (2015): 83–96. https://www.ncbi.nlm.nih.gov/pmc/articles/PMC4378297/.

199. Ibid.

200. Menigoz, Wendy, Tracy T. Latz, Robin A. Ely, Cimone Kamei, Gregory Melvin, and Drew Sinatra. "Integrative and Lifestyle Medicine Strategies Should Include Earthing (Grounding): Review of Research Evidence and Clinical Observations." *Explore* 16, no. 3 (2020): 152–160. https://pubmed.ncbi.nlm.nih.gov/31831261/.

201. Sinatra S. T., G. Chevalier, and D. Sinatra. "Vitamin G. Grounding as Energetic Nutrition and Its Role in Oxidative Defense and Cardiovascular Disease." In *Nutritional and Integrative Strategies in Cardiovascular Medicine*, edited by S. T. Sinatra and M. C. Houston. CRC Press, 2022, 359–368; Sinatra S.T., J. L. Oschman, G. Chevalier, and D. Sinatra.. "Electric Nutrition: The Surprising Health and Healing Benefits of Biological Grounding (Earthing)." *Alternative Therapies in Health and Medicine* 23, no. 5 2017): 8–16. https://pubmed.ncbi.nlm.nih.gov/28987038/

202. Menigoz, Wendy, Tracy T. Latz, Robin A. Ely, Cimone Kamei, Gregory Melvin, and Drew Sinatra. "Integrative and Lifestyle Medicine Strategies Should Include Earthing (Grounding): Review of Research Evidence and Clinical Observations." *Explore* 16, no. 3 (2020): 152–160. https://pubmed.ncbi.nlm.nih.gov/31831261/.

203. Oschman, James L., Gaétan Chevalier, and Richard Brown. "The Effects of Grounding (Earthing) on Inflammation, the Immune Response, Wound Healing, and Prevention and Treatment of Chronic Inflammatory and Autoimmune Diseases." *Journal of Inflammation Research* 8 (2015): 83–96. https://www.ncbi.nlm.nih.gov/pmc/articles/PMC4378297/.

204. Ibid.

205. Leigh, Charlotte, Maurice Faigenblum, Peter Fine, Robert Blizard, and Albert Leung. "General Dental Practitioners' Knowledge and Opinions of Snoring and Sleep-Related Breathing Disorders." *British Dental Journal* 231, no. 9 (2021): 569–574. https://www.ncbi.nlm.nih.gov/pmc/articles/PMC8589666/.

206. Lin, Chien-Hung, Shih-Ting Tseng, Yao-Chung Chuang, Chun-En Kuo, and Nai-Ching Chen. "Grounding the Body Improves Sleep Quality in Patients with Mild Alzheimer's Disease: A Pilot Study." *Healthcare* 10, no. 3 (2022): 581. https://pubmed.ncbi.nlm.nih.gov/35327058/.

207. Sokal, Karol and Pawel Sokal. "Earthing the Human Body Influences Physiologic Processes." *Journal of Alternative and Complementary Medicine* 17, no. 4 (2011): 301–308. https://pubmed.ncbi.nlm.nih.gov/21469913/.

208. "Electrolytes: Types, Purpose & Normal Levels." Cleveland Clinic. 2021. https://my .clevelandclinic.org/health/diagnostics/21790-electrolytes.

209. "Electrolyte Imbalance: Types, Symptoms, Causes & Treatment." Cleveland Clinic. 2022. https://my.clevelandclinic.org/health/symptoms/24019-electrolyte-imbalance.

210. Munch, Daniel. "Over 140,000 Farms Lost in 5 Years." FarmWeek Now. March 7, 2024. https://www.farmweeknow.com/news/extra_intel/over-140-000-farms-lost-in -5-years/article_01a2a756-dc9b-11ee-9290-0baafae0f70f.html.

211. HusFarm. "The Impact of Monocropping on Soil Biodiversity and How to Counteract It." *HusFarm.com.* Accessed August 16, 2024. https://husfarm.com/impact -monocropping-soil-biodiversity.

212. McDaniel, M. D., L. K. Tiemann, and A. S. Grandy. "Does Agricultural Crop Diversity Enhance Soil Microbial Biomass and Organic Matter Dynamics? A Meta-Analysis." *Ecological Applications* 24, no. 3 (2014): 560–70. https://doi.org/10.1890/13 -0616.1.

213. "How Our Food System Affects Public Health." FoodPrint. February 28, 2024. https://foodprint.org/issues/how-our-food-system-affects-public-health/.

214. Gunnars, Kris. "Why High-Fructose Corn Syrup Is Bad for You." Healthline. Last modified June 8, 2023. Accessed November 5, 2024. https://www.healthline.com /nutrition/why-high-fructose-corn-syrup-is-bad#3-Increases-your-risk-of-obesity -and-weight-gain.

215. Radak, Zsolt, Zhongfu Zhao, Erika Koltai, Hideki Ohno, and Mustafa Atalay. "Oxygen Consumption and Usage during Physical Exercise: The Balance Between Oxidative Stress and Ros-Dependent Adaptive Signaling." *Antioxidants & Redox Signaling* 18, no. 10 (2013): 1208–1246. https://www.ncbi.nlm.nih.gov/pmc/articles /PMC3579386/.

216. "Functions of Blood: Transport around the Body." NHS Blood Donation. Accessed May 20, 2024. https://www.blood.co.uk/news-and-campaigns/the-donor/latest -stories/functions-of-blood-transport-around-the-body/.

217. Alberts, Bruce. "How Cells Obtain Energy from Food." *Molecular Biology of the Cell*, 4th edition. January 1, 1970. https://www.ncbi.nlm.nih.gov/books/NBK26882/.

218. Zenewicz, Lauren A. "Oxygen Levels and Immunological Studies." *Frontiers in Immunology* 8 (2017_: 324. https://www.ncbi.nlm.nih.gov/pmc/articles/PMC5359232/.

219. Pittman, Roland N. "The Circulatory System and Oxygen Transport." *Regulation of Tissue Oxygenation*, January 1, 1970. https://www.ncbi.nlm.nih.gov/books /NBK54112/; Katz, A. and K. Sahlin. "Regulation of Lactic Acid Production during Exercise." *Journal of Applied Physiology* 65, no. 2 (1988): 509–519. https://pubmed .ncbi.nlm.nih.gov/3049511/.

220. Alberts, Bruce. "How Cells Obtain Energy from Food." *Molecular Biology of the Cell*, 4th edition. January 1, 1970. https://www.ncbi.nlm.nih.gov/books/NBK26882/.

221. Merritt, Edward K. "Why Is It So Hard to Lose Fat? Because It Has to Get Out Through Your Nose! An Exercise Physiology Laboratory on Oxygen Consumption, Metabolism, and Weight Loss." *Advances in Physiology Education* 45, no. 3 (2021): 599–606. https://pubmed.ncbi.nlm.nih.gov/34379483/.

222. Pittman, Roland N. "The Circulatory System and Oxygen Transport." *Regulation of Tissue Oxygenation*, January 1, 1970. https://www.ncbi.nlm.nih.gov/books /NBK54112/; Katz, A. and K. Sahlin. "Regulation of Lactic Acid Production during Exercise." *Journal of Applied Physiology* 65, no. 2 (1988): 509–519. https://pubmed .ncbi.nlm.nih.gov/3049511/.

223. Castilla, Diego M., Zhao-Jun Liu, and Omaida C. Velazquez. "Oxygen: Implications for Wound Healing." *Advances in Wound Care* 1, no. 6 (2012): 225–230. https://www .ncbi.nlm.nih.gov/pmc/articles/PMC3625368/.

224. Shields, Hazel J., Annika Traa, and Jeremy M. Van Raamsdonk. "Beneficial and Detrimental Effects of Reactive Oxygen Species on Lifespan: A Comprehensive Review of Comparative and Experimental Studies." *Frontiers in Cell and Developmental Biology* 9 (2021): 628157. https://www.ncbi.nlm.nih.gov/pmc/articles/PMC7905231/.

225. Imtiyaz, Hongxia Z. and M. Celeste Simon. "Hypoxia-Inducible Factors as Essential Regulators of Inflammation." *Current Topics in Microbiology and Immunology* 345 (2010): 105–120. https://www.ncbi.nlm.nih.gov/pmc/articles/PMC3144567/.

226. Li, Xiaolu, Yanyan Yang, Bei Zhang, Xiaotong Lin, Xiuxiu Fu, Yi An, Yulin Zou, Jian-Xun Wang, Zhibin Wang, and Tao Yu. "Lactate Metabolism in Human Health and Disease." *Signal Transduction and Targeted Therapy* 7 (2022): 305. https://www .ncbi.nlm.nih.gov/pmc/articles/PMC9434547/.

227. Michiels, Carine. "Physiological and Pathological Responses to Hypoxia." *The American Journal of Pathology* 164, no. 6 (2004): 1875–1882. https://www.ncbi.nlm.nih .gov/pmc/articles/PMC1615763/.

228. Semenza, Gregg L. "Hypoxia-Inducible Factors in Physiology and Medicine." *Cell* 148, no. 3 (2012): 399–408. https://doi.org/10.1016/j.cell.2012.01.021.

229. Castillo-Rodríguez, R. A., C. Trejo-Solís, A. Cabrera-Cano, S. Gómez-Manzo, and V. M. Dávila-Borja. "Hypoxia as a Modulator of Inflammation and Immune Response in Cancer." *Cancers (Basel)* 14, no. 9 (May 4, 2022): 2291. https://doi.org /10.3390/cancers14092291.

230. Flaherty, Julie. "The Body on Fire." *Tufts Now*. October 5, 2012. https://now.tufts .edu/2012/10/05/body-fire.

231. Fuhrman, Joel. "The Hidden Dangers of Fast and Processed Food." *American Journal of Lifestyle Medicine* 12, no. 5 (2018): 375–381. https://www.ncbi.nlm.nih.gov/pmc /articles/PMC6146358/.

232. "The Truth About Fats: The Good, the Bad, and the In-Between." Harvard Health. April 12, 2022. https://www.health.harvard.edu/staying-healthy/the-truth-about-fats -bad-and-good.

233. Richard-Eaglin, Angela, and Benjamin A. Smallheer. "Immunosuppressive/Autoimmune Disorders." *Nursing Clinics of North America* 53, no. 3 (2018): 319–334. https:// pubmed.ncbi.nlm.nih.gov/30099999/.

234. You, Yanwei, Yuquan Chen, Wen Fang, Xingtian Li, Rui Wang, Jianxiu Liu, and Xindong Ma. "The Association Between Sedentary Behavior, Exercise, and Sleep Disturbance: A Mediation Analysis of Inflammatory Biomarkers." *Frontiers in Immunology* 13 (2023): 1080782. https://www.ncbi.nlm.nih.gov/pmc/articles/PMC9880546/.

235. Chung, Hae Young, Dae Hyun Kim, Eun Kyeong Lee, Ki Wung Chung, Sangwoon Chung, Bonggi Lee, Arnold Y. Seo, et al. "Redefining Chronic Inflammation in Aging and Age-Related Diseases: Proposal of the Senoinflammation Concept." *Aging and Disease* 10, no. 2 (2019): 367–382. https://www.ncbi.nlm.nih.gov/pmc/articles /PMC6457053/.

236. Ernst, Joel Đ. "Mechanisms of M. tuberculosis Immune Evasion as Challenges to TB Vaccine Design." *Cell Host & Microbe* 24, no. 1 (July 11, 2018): 34–42. https://doi .org/10.1016/j.chom.2018.06.004. PMID: 30001523; PMCID: PMC6482466.

237. Shetty, Shilpa S., D. Deepthi, S. Harshitha, Shipra Sonkusare, Prashanth B. Naik, Kumari N. Suchetha, and Harishkumar Madhyastha. "Environmental Pollutants and Their Effects on Human Health." *Heliyon* 9, no. 9 (2023): e19496. https://www .ncbi.nlm.nih.gov/pmc/articles/PMC10472068/.

238. Ellulu, Mohammed S., Ismail Patimah, Huzwah Khaza'ai, Asmah Rahmat, and Yehia Abed. "Obesity and Inflammation: The Linking Mechanism and the Complications." *Archives of Medical Science* 13, no. 4 (2017): 851–863. https://www.ncbi.nlm .nih.gov/pmc/articles/PMC5507106/.

239. Morey, Jennifer N., Ian A. Boggero, April B. Scott, and Suzanne C. Segerstrom. "Current Directions in Stress and Human Immune Function." *Current Opinion in Psychology* 5 (2015): 13–17. https://www.ncbi.nlm.nih.gov/pmc/articles/PMC4465119/.

240. Pahwa, Roma, Amandeep Goyal, and Ishwarlal Jialal. "Chronic Inflammation." StatPearls. August 7, 2023. https://www.ncbi.nlm.nih.gov/books/NBK493173/.

241. "Sleep Health." National Heart Lung and Blood Institute. Accessed May 20, 2024. https://www.nhlbi.nih.gov/health-topics/education-and-awareness/sleep-health.

242. Mitra A. K., A. R. Bhuiyan, and E. A. Jones. "Association and Risk Factors for Obstructive Sleep Apnea and Cardiovascular Diseases: A Systematic Review." *Diseases* 9, no. 4 (2021): 88. doi: 10.3390/diseases9040088. PMID: 34940026; PMCID: PMC8700568.

243. Yeghiazarians, Yerem, Hani Jneid, Jeremy R. Tietjens, Susan Redline, Devin L. Brown, Nabil El-Sherif, Reena Mehra, Biykem Bozkurt, Chiadi Ericson Ndumele, and Virend K. Somers. "Obstructive Sleep Apnea and Cardiovascular Disease: A Scientific Statement From the American Heart Association." *Circulation* 144, no. 3(2021): e56 - e67. https://www.ahajournals.org/doi/full/10.1161/CIR .0000000000000988.

244. Ibid.

245. Benjamin, Emelia J., Michael J. Blaha, Stephanie E. Chiuve, Mary Cushman, Sandeep R. Das, Rajat Deo, Sarah D. de Ferranti, et al. "Heart Disease and Stroke Statistics-2017 Update: A Report from the American Heart Association." *Circulation* 135, no. 10 (2017): e146–e603. https://www.ncbi.nlm.nih.gov/pmc/articles /PMC5408160/.

246. Lee, Yun-Gi, Pureun-Haneul Lee, Seon-Muk Choi, Min-Hyeok An, and An-Soo Jang. "Effects of Air Pollutants on Airway Diseases." *International Journal of Environmental Research and Public Health* 18, no. 18 (2021): 9905. https://www.ncbi.nlm .nih.gov/pmc/articles/PMC8465980/.

247. Leontjevaite, Kristina. "Unveiling the Hidden Role of Plants in Regulating Air Quality." Earth.Org. March 30, 2024. https://earth.org/unveiling-plants-hidden-air -quality-role/.

248. Ritchie, Hannah and Max Roser. "Indoor Air Pollution." Our World in Data. March 15, 2024. https://ourworldindata.org/indoor-air-pollution.

249. "Why Indoor Air Quality Is Important to Schools." EPA. Accessed May 20, 2024. https://www.epa.gov/iaq-schools/why-indoor-air-quality-important-schools; "What Are the Trends in Indoor Air Quality and Their Effects on Human Health?" EPA. Accessed May 20, 2024. https://www.epa.gov/report-environment/indoor-air-quality #note1.

250. Popkin, Barry M., Karen E. D'Anci, and Irwin H. Rosenberg. "Water, Hydration, and Health." *Nutrition Reviews* 68, no. 8 (2010): 439–58. https://doi.org/10.1111 /j.1753-4887.2010.00304.x.

251. Kravitz, Len. "Water: The Science of Nature's Most Important Nutrient." UNM. Accessed May 22, 2024. https://www.unm.edu/~lkravitz/Article%20folder/Water UNM.html.

252. Palsdottir, Hrefna. "Drink 8 Glasses of Water a Day: Fact or Fiction?" *Healthline*. November 20, 2023. https://www.healthline.com/nutrition/8-glasses-of-water-per -day.

253. Ibid.

254. Mehta, Ravi and Rui (Juliet) Zhu. "Blue or Red? Exploring the Effect of Color on Cognitive Task Performances." *Science* 323, no. 5918 (2009): 1226–1229. https:// www.science.org/doi/10.1126/science.1169144.

255. Ratcliffe, Eleanor. "Sound and Soundscape in Restorative Natural Environments: A Narrative Literature Review." *Frontiers in Psychology* 12 (2021): 570563. https://www .ncbi.nlm.nih.gov/pmc/articles/PMC8107214/.

256. Team, The Cell Health. "The Science behind Ocean Negative Ions and Their Health Benefits." *Cell Health News*. April 17, 2023. https://cellhealthnews.com/articles/the -science-behind-ocean-negative-ions/.

257. Perez, Vanessa, Dominik D. Alexander, and William H Bailey. "Air Ions and Mood Outcomes: A Review and Meta-Analysis." *BMC Psychiatry* 13, article 29 (2013). https://bmcpsychiatry.biomedcentral.com/articles/10.1186/1471-244X-13-29.

258. Singh, Anubhav, Anuj Sharma, Rohit K. Verma, Rushikesh L. Chopade, Pritam P. Pandit, Varad Nagar, Vinay Aseri, et al. "Heavy Metal Contamination of Water and Their Toxic Effect on Living Organisms." IntechOpen. June 15, 2022. https://www .intechopen.com/chapters/82246.

259. "Globally, 3 Billion People at Health Risk Due to Scarce Data on Water Quality." UNEP. March 19, 2021. https://www.unep.org/news-and-stories/story/globally -3-billion-people-health-risk-due-scarce-data-water-quality.

260. Stoiber, Tasha. "EWG Survey: At Least 50 Percent of People Surveyed Think Tap Water Is Unsafe." Environmental Working Group. August 11, 2022. https://www .ewg.org/research/ewg-survey-least-50-percent-people-surveyed-think-tap-water -unsafe.

261. Communications and Publishing. "Tap Water Study Detects PFAS 'Forever Chemicals' Across the US: U.S. Geological Survey." U.S. Geological Survey. July 5, 2023. https://www.usgs.gov/news/national-news-release/tap-water-study-detects-pfas -forever-chemicals-across-us.

262. Ibid.

263. "Potential Health Effects of PFAS Chemicals." Centers for Disease Control and Prevention. January 18, 2024. https://www.atsdr.cdc.gov/pfas/health-effects/index .html.

264. Razgaitis, Richard. "Council Post: Growth Trends in the Water Purification Industry." *Forbes*. November 16, 2023. https://www.forbes.com/sites/forbesbusinesscouncil /2023/11/15/growth-trends-in-the-water-purification-industry/?sh=395b8a827a1c.

265. Johnston, N. R. and S. A. Strobel. "Principles of Fluoride Toxicity and the Cellular Response: A Review." *Archives of Toxicology* 94, no. 4 (April 2020): 1051–1069. https://doi.org/10.1007/s00204-020-02687-5.

266. Iamandii, I., L. De Pasquale, M. E. Giannone, F. Veneri, L. Generali, U. Consolo, L. S. Birnbaum, J. Castenmiller, T. I. Halldorsson, T. Filippini, and M. Vinceti. "Does Fluoride Exposure Affect Thyroid Function? A Systematic Review and Dose-Response Meta-Analysis." *Environmental Research* 242 (2024): 117759. https:// doi.org/10.1016/j.envres.2023.117759.

267. Żwierełło, W., A. Maruszewska, M. Skórka-Majewicz, and I. Gutowska. "Fluoride in the Central Nervous System and Its Potential Influence on the Development and Invasiveness of Brain Tumours—A Research Hypothesis." *International Journal of Molecular Sciences* 24, no. 2 (2023): 1558. https://doi.org/10.3390/ijms24021558.

268. Goodman, C., M. Hall, R. Green, R. Hornung, E. A. Martinez-Mier, B. Lanphear, and C. Till. "Maternal Fluoride Exposure, Fertility, and Birth Outcomes: The MIREC Cohort." *Environmental Advances* 7 (2022): 100135. https://doi.org/10.1016 /j.envadv.2021.100135.

269. Veneri, Federica, Marco Vinceti, Luigi Generali, Maria Edvige Giannone, Elena Mazzoleni, Linda S. Birnbaum, Ugo Consolo, and Tommaso Filippini. "Fluoride Exposure and Cognitive Neurodevelopment: Systematic Review and Dose-Response Meta-Analysis." *Environmental Research* 221 (2023): 115239. https://doi.org/10.1016 /j.envres.2023.115239.

270. Butera, A., S. Gallo, M. Pascadopoli, M. A. Montasser, M. H. Abd El Latief, G. G. Modica, and A. Scribante. "Home Oral Care with Biomimetic Hydroxyapatite vs. Conventional Fluoridated Toothpaste for the Remineralization and Desensitizing of White Spot Lesions: Randomized Clinical Trial." *International Journal of Environmental Research and Public Health* 19, no. 14 (2022): 8676. https://doi.org/10.3390 /ijerph19148676.

271. Kamalapriya, V., R. Mani, V. Venkatesh, S. Kunhikannan, and V. S. Ganesh. "The Role of Low Mineral Water Consumption in Reducing the Mineral Density of Bones and Teeth: A Narrative Review." *Cureus* 15, no. 11 (2023): e49119. https://doi.org/10 .7759/cureus.49119.

272. Peake, Jonathan M., Llion A. Roberts, Vandre C. Figueiredo, Ingrid Egner, Simone Krog, Sigve N. Aas, Katsuhiko Suzuki, et al. "The Effects of Cold Water Immersion

and Active Recovery on Inflammation and Cell Stress Responses in Human Skeletal Muscle after Resistance Exercise." *The Journal of Physiology* 595, no. 3 (2016): 695–711. https://www.ncbi.nlm.nih.gov/pmc/articles/PMC5285720/.

273. Bleakley, Chris, Suzanne McDonough, Evie Gardner, G. David Baxter, J. Ty Hopkins, and Gareth W. Davison. "Cold-Water Immersion (Cryotherapy) for Preventing and Treating Muscle Soreness After Exercise." *The Cochrane Database of Systematic Reviews* no. 3 (2012): CD008262. https://www.ncbi.nlm.nih.gov/pmc/articles/PMC6492480/.

274. Team, The Cell Health. "The Science behind Ocean Negative Ions and Their Health Benefits." Cell Health News. April 17, 2023. https://cellhealthnews.com/articles/the-science-behind-ocean-negative-ions/.

275. "The Safe Mercury Amalgam Removal Technique (SMART)." IAOMT. December 12, 2023. https://iaomt.org/resources/safe-removal-amalgam-fillings/.

276. Houghton-Rahrig, Lori D., Debra L. Schutte, Alexander von Eye, Jenifer I. Fenton, Barbara A. Given, and Norman G. Hord. "Exploration of a Symptoms Experience in People with Obesity-Related Nonalcoholic Fatty Liver Disease." *Nursing Outlook* 61, no. 4 (2013): 242–251.e2. https://www.ncbi.nlm.nih.gov/pmc/articles/PMC3799949/.

277. Samtiya, Meenakshi, Rotimi E. Aluko, and Thakur Dhewa. "Plant Food Antinutritional Factors and Their Reduction Strategies: An Overview." *Food Production, Processing and Nutrition* 2, no. 6 (2020). https://doi.org/10.1186/s43014-020-0020-5.

INDEX

ABOUT THE AUTHOR

Dr. Michelle Jorgensen's journey began when she became seriously ill due to mercury exposure from practicing traditional dentistry. This life-changing experience led her to rethink not only the dental care she provided but also health care as a whole. She became a Board-Certified Holistic Health Practitioner, and seamlessly integrated medicine and dentistry into a new model at her whole health–based practice, Total Care Dental and Wellness. Inspired by a desire to share her own approach to living well, she founded Living Well with Dr. Michelle and the new Cell Well Center, helping people navigate their journey to Living Well. Through these platforms and centers, she provides nature- and science-backed products, information, and practical solutions to help people navigate the overwhelming amount of wellness information available today and reclaim their ability to care for their own health. In addition to being a busy mother and grandmother, she loves teaching, writing, cooking, and gardening, and firmly believes the earth provides everything we need to live well.